A GUIDE TO INTERPRETATION OF
HEMODYNAMIC DATA
IN THE CORONARY CARE UNIT

A GUIDE TO INTERPRETATION OF
HEMODYNAMIC DATA
IN THE CORONARY CARE UNIT

SCOTT W. SHARKEY, M.D.

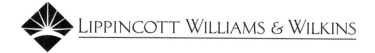

Acquisitions Editor: Ruth Weinberg
Developmental Editor: Renee Gagliardi
Manufacturing Manager: Dennis Teston
Production Manager: Lawrence Bernstein
Production Editor: Christina Zingone
Cover Designer: MaryAnn M. Brower
Indexer: Susan Lohmeyer
Compositor: MaryAnn M. Brower
Printer: Maple Press

Printed in the United States of America

9 8 7 6 5 4 3 2

Library of Congress Cataloging-in-Publication Data
Sharkey, Scott W.
    A guide to interpretation of hemodynamic data in the coronary care unit / Scott W. Sharkey.
        p.   cm.
    Includes bibliographical references and index.
    ISBN 0-397-58782-1
    1. Cardiac intensive care.   2. Hemodynamic monitoring.   3. Coronary care units.   I. Title.
    [DNLM: 1. Heart Diseases–physiopathology.   2. Ventricular Function–physiology.   3. Hemodynamics–physiology.   4. Monitoring, Physiologic.   WG 210 S531g 1997]
    RC684.I56S53   1997
    616.1'2028–dc21
    DNLM/DLC
For Library of Congress

To PJS

"You are very special"

CONTENTS

ACKNOWLEDGMENTS

This manual reflects the hard work of many individuals. Dr. Harold Osher at the Maine Medical Center encouraged my interest in cardiology. Dr. Yang Wang and Dr. Richard Asinger at the University of Minnesota taught me many principles of hemodynamic monitoring. Dr. Asinger has a natural ability to relate basic physiologic principles to the evaluation and management of the patient. Dr. Morrison Hodges at the University of Minnesota encouraged me to write about bedside hemodynamic monitoring. He had the foresight to install a multi-channel recorder in our Coronary Care Unit which allowed me to make many of the recordings shown in this manual. Dr. James Leatherman taught me much about respiration and hemodynamic monitoring. I am grateful to Dr. Jeremy Swan for taking the time to critique the manuscript and figures. His suggestions greatly improved this manual.

The countless revisions of the text for this manual are the results of Rosie Robinson's skilled efforts. Maureen Adams helped me to prepare many of the figures. Tom Buchanan and Mary Greenwood helped with recordings made in the cardiac catheterization laboratory. This manual was produced and designed by MaryAnn Brower. She is a wizard with the Apple computer. Ruth Weinberg was the editor for this project. She provided encouragement and perspective. Many of her suggestions have been incorporated into this book.

The staff in the George E. Fahr Coronary Care Unit at the Hennepin County Medical Center are the heart and soul of this manual. Sheila Elledge, RN, has fostered an environment which stimulates research and education. The nursing staff is responsible for the exceptional quality of the hemodynamic monitoring in our Coronary Care Unit.

INTRODUCTION

In 1970, the pulmonary artery catheter was introduced into clinical medicine by Drs. William Ganz and Jeremy Swan. This catheter is now commonly referred to as the Swan-Ganz catheter. With the introduction of the pulmonary artery catheter, physicians were able to perform hemodynamic monitoring at the bedside in critically ill patients. Early research efforts using the pulmonary artery catheter focused on acute myocardial infarction and its complications.

Bedside hemodynamic monitoring expanded rapidly to encompass the coronary care unit, the medical intensive care unit, the surgical intensive care unit, and the operating room. Currently, hemodynamic monitoring is performed by an entire spectrum of physicians. Anesthesiologists, trauma surgeons, pulmonologists, nephrologists, critical care specialists, and cardiologists all commonly perform bedside hemodynamic monitoring.

During training, physicians are tempted to focus on learning procedure related skills. It is thrilling to successfully puncture the subclavian vein on the first attempt. Learning invasive techniques is an important aspect of providing high quality patient care. Nonetheless, it is the interpretation of hemodynamic data which requires the most study. Bedside hemodynamic monitoring involves far more than measuring the wedge pressure and the cardiac output.

The physiologic principles presented in this book are immutable. An investment in time to learn these principles will reap many rewards. Who can deny the immense satisfaction of diagnosing pericardial tamponade by recognizing the absent Y descent on a right atrial pressure tracing. It is my hope that this book will provide a platform for students, residents, and fellows to study and understand hemodynamic monitoring in the coronary care unit. The well being of the patient rests on the skill and knowledge of their physician.

NORMAL PHYSIOLOGY

It is not possible to understand hemodynamic monitoring in the coronary care unit without thorough study of normal cardiovascular physiology. Myocardial contraction is ultimately initiated by an electrical stimulus. An understanding of the relation between the electrocardiographic and hemodynamic events is therefore essential. The physician must know the sequence of pressure events in each of the four cardiac chambers as well as the pulmonary artery and the aorta. The effects of breathing must be considered since respiration itself influences the intracardiac pressure and blood flow. It is equally important to know the proper technique of pressure measurement; calibration, zeroing, and transducer placement are crucial details. Finally, the physician must know the design of the pulmonary artery catheter and the principles of the wedge pressure measurement.

Pressure Measurement

Measurement of the intracardiac pressure is fundamental to hemodynamic monitoring. Intracardiac pressure is measured in mmHg (relative to atmospheric pressure) and normal values are reported referenced to atmosphere.[1] Although atmospheric pressure varies with time and altitude, this is not usually clinically important. Except at the time of open cardiac surgery, the heart is not exposed to the atmosphere. Instead, it is surrounded by the pericardium and the thorax. Intracardiac pressure measurements therefore are subject to the influence of the blood volume in the cardiac chambers, the pericardial pressure, and the intrathoracic pressure. In normal individuals, the intrapericardial pressure and the intrathoracic pressure are equal and subatmospheric (i.e. negative).[2] The transmural (distending) pressure is a measure of the force which stretches the myofibrils.[2] This is commonly referred to as the preload. To determine the transmural pressure within a cardiac chamber, the intrathoracic pressure must be subtracted from the intracardiac pressure measurement. For example, in an individual with a right atrial pressure measurement of +5 mmHg (referenced to atmosphere) and an intrathoracic pressure measurement of -4 mmHg (referenced to atmosphere) the right atrial transmural pressure would be 5 - (-4) = +9 mmHg. If the intrathoracic pressure was +4 mmHg instead of -4 mmHg, the transmural pressure would be 5 - (+4) = +1 mmHg. The intrathoracic pressure cannot be easily measured and it is often ignored when interpreting intracardiac pressure data. This approach works in most instances because the intrathoracic pressure is usually negligible. In patients with significant lung disease or respiratory distress, the intrathoracic pressure will dominate the intracardiac pressure measurement. In this situation, an attempt should be made to subtract the intrathoracic pressure from the intracardiac pressure to yield the transmural pressure. This is discussed further in Chapter 2. Intrathoracic pressure is usually measured in cm H_2O and must be converted to mmHg before subtracting it from the intracardiac pressure. The conversion formula is:

cm H_2O x 0.74 = mmHg

(1 mmHg = 1.36 cm H_2O)

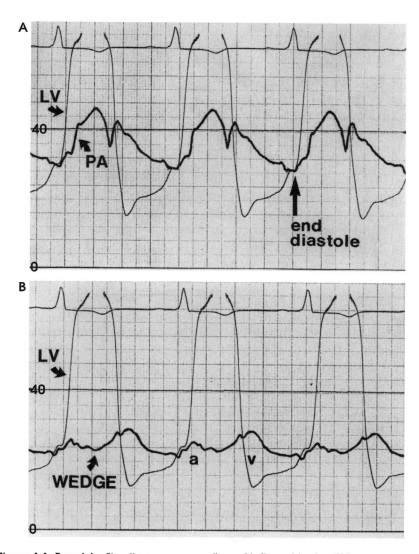

Figure 1.1 Panel A: Simultaneous recording of left ventricular (**LV**) pressure and pulmonary artery (**PA**) pressure made in the Cardiac Catheterization Laboratory. At end diastole (**arrow**), the pulmonary artery pressure and the left ventricular pressure are equal (28 mmHg) in this patient with normal pulmonary vascular resistance.
Panel B: Simultaneous recording of LV pressure and wedge pressure from the same patient. The mean wedge pressure (25 mmHg), the pulmonary artery diastolic pressure (28 mmHg) and the left ventricular end diastolic pressure (28 mmHg) are approximately equal (pressure difference ≤ 5 mmHg).
Scale = 0-40 mmHg; Paper speed = 50 mm/sec.

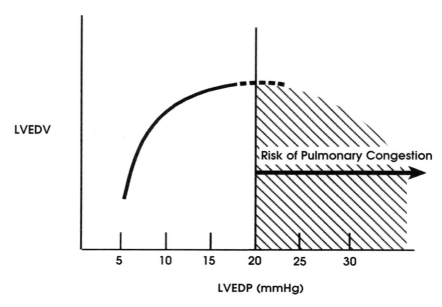

Figure 1.2 Relation between left ventricular end-diastolic pressure (**LVEDP**) and left ventricular end-diastolic volume (**LVEDV**). In normal hearts the left ventricular end-diastolic pressure is low (10-12 mmHg). Optimal left ventricular filling occurs at a hydrostatic pressure well below that associated with pulmonary congestion.

Left Ventricular Pressure
Normal left ventricular pressures are[1]:

Systolic	100-140 mmHg
End-diastolic	3-12 mmHg

Left ventricular pressure cannot be measured directly using bedside monitoring techniques. Nonetheless, it is possible to accurately estimate the left ventricular pressure in the following way:

- The left ventricular systolic pressure equals the aortic systolic pressure in the absence of left ventricular outflow obstruction.

- The left ventricular end-diastolic pressure equals the mean wedge pressure in the absence of mitral valve disease.

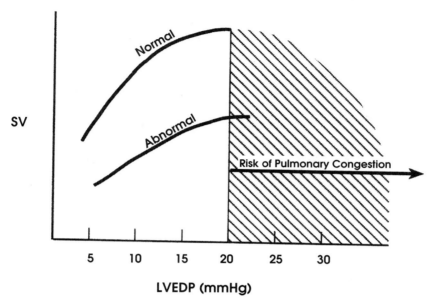

Figure 1.3 Relation between left ventricular end-diastolic pressure (**LVEDP**) and stroke volume (**SV**) in normal and abnormal hearts. In abnormal hearts, the response of stroke volume to an increase in the LVEDP is diminished. With disease, optimal filling pressures occurs at an LVEDP of 20-25 mmHg.

The end of left ventricular diastole coincides with the onset of the electrocardiographic QRS complex. The left ventricular end-diastolic pressure is a key physiologic parameter *(Figure 1.1)*.[3-5] This is commonly referred to as the left ventricular filling pressure reflecting its use as an estimate of left ventricular filling volume *(Figure 1.2)*. Measurement of the left ventricular end-diastolic pressure allows the clinician to use the Frank-Starling principle to assess and manipulate left ventricular performance *(Figure 1.3)*.[6] Myocardial or pericardial disease significantly alters the relation between left ventricular end-diastolic pressure and volume.[6] As a rule, cardiac disease causes a decrease in compliance; the result is a higher filling pressure to achieve the same degree of filling volume. At the same time, cardiac disease diminishes the response of left ventricular performance to an increase in the end-

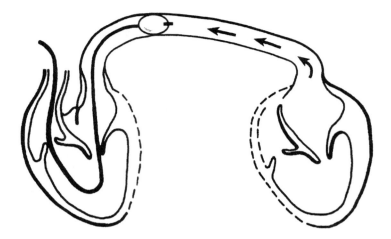

Figure 1.4 Schematic diagram depicting the principle of the wedge pressure measurements. Inflation of the pulmonary artery catheter balloon obstructs blood flow in a segment of pulmonary artery. A blood filled channel connects the distal catheter lumen with the left atrium. Left atrial pressure waves are transmitted retrograde through this channel to the catheter lumen and then to the pressure transducer.

diastolic pressure[6] *(Figure 1.3)*. The left ventricular end-diastolic pressure for a normal heart is 3-12 mmHg.[1] With left ventricular disease (acute myocardial infarction, cardiomyopathy), the optimal filling pressure increases to 20-25 mmHg.[7] The need to maintain a higher left ventricular filling pressure comes with a price since an increase in the diastolic pressure eventually leads to pulmonary congestion.

Wedge Pressure
The wedge pressure waveform is an indirect recording of left atrial mechanical events.[8-10] Knowledge of the left atrial pressure provides an estimate of both the left ventricular end-diastolic pressure and the hydrostatic pressure in the pulmonary capillary bed. Inflation of the balloon at the tip of the pulmonary artery catheter obstructs a pulmonary artery segment creating a fluid-filled "window" into the left atrium *(Figure 1.4)*. Left atrial mechanical

events are transmitted retrogradely through the pulmonary vascular bed, the distal catheter lumen, and then to the transducer *(Figure 1.5)*. Retrograde transmission of the left atrial pressure events smoothes (dampens) the A and V waves and the X and Y descents.[1] The C wave is often invisible in the wedge waveform because of damping. The retrograde transmission also introduces a significant delay between electrocardiographic and mechanical events.

The normal mean wedge pressure is 2-12 mmHg and is twice the mean right atrial pressure.[1] The wedge pressure A wave follows the electrocardiographic P wave by $\geq$ 200 msec *(Figure 1.5)*. The A wave represents left atrial systole. The A wave magnitude is increased in conditions such as mitral stenosis and left ventricular noncompliance. The C wave is caused by closure of the mitral valve and marks the onset of left ventricular systole. The C wave is visible in the left atrial pressure recording but is often not seen in the wedge pressure waveform because of damping. The V wave represents venous filling of the left atrium when left ventricular systole has closed the mitral valve. The peak of the V wave marks the end of left ventricular systole. In some normal patients, the V wave is the dominant positive wave in the wedge pressure waveform.[11] Left atrial volume overload from mitral regurgitation or a ventricular septal defect will magnify the V wave. The peak of the V wave occurs after the T wave of the electrocardiogram and is noticeably later than the pulmonary artery systolic wave *(Figure 1.5)*. This difference in timing becomes important when interpreting hemodynamic data from patients with a giant V wave *(Chapter 5)*.

The X and Y descents follow the A and V waves respectively *(Figure 1.5)*. The X descent represents left atrial relaxation combined with the sudden downward motion of the atrioventricular junction during early left ventricular systole. Mitral regurgitation can attenuate or obliterate the X descent. The Y descent is caused by the rapid exit of blood from the left atrium into the left ventricle at the moment of mitral valve opening. The Y descent marks the onset of left ventricular diastole. The Y descent is

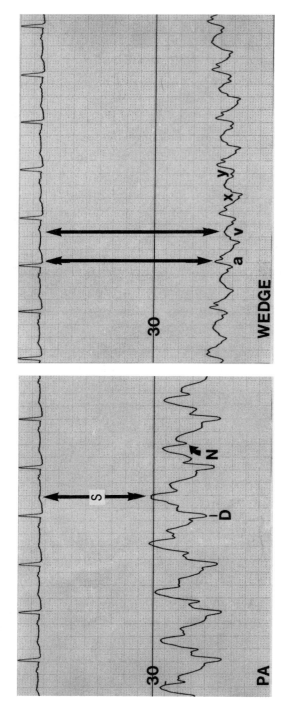

Figure 1.5 Normal pulmonary artery (**PA**) and wedge pressure waveforms. Sinus rhythm is present. The pulmonary artery pressure (left) is 31/19 mmHg. The pulse pressure is 12 mmHg. The pulmonary artery systolic wave (**S**) coincides with the T wave of the electrocardiogram. The dicrotic notch (**N**) marks pulmonic valve closure. Its crisp character signifies a high quality recording. The mean wedge pressure (right) is 15 mmHg at end-expiration. The pulmonary artery diastolic pressure (**D**) is within 5 mmHg of the mean wedge pressure in this patient with normal pulmonary vascular resistance. The A (**a**) and V (**v**) waves of the wedge pressure waveform are similar in amplitude. Compare the timing of the wedge pressure A and V waves here with the right atrial pressure A and V waves from the same patient (*Figure 1.11*). Note also that the wedge pressure V wave occurs significantly later in time than the pulmonary artery systolic wave. Scale = 0-30 mmHg; Paper speed = 25 mm/sec.

blunted with mitral stenosis. Coincident with the X and Y descents, there is a surge of pulmonary venous return to the left atrium.

Clinical Use of the Wedge Pressure Measurement[12]

The wedge pressure is used clinically in the following ways:

- To assess the adequacy of left ventricular filling.

- To determine the hydrostatic pressure in the pulmonary veins.

The mean wedge pressure is usually an accurate measure of the left ventricular end-diastolic pressure *(Figure 1.1)*.[12,13] Using the Frank-Starling principle, the mean wedge pressure can be manipulated (for example, volume infusion or diuretic administration) to achieve an optimal left ventricular stroke volume. While the optimal left ventricular end-diastolic pressure for a damaged left ventricle is 20-25 mmHg, the optimal wedge pressure for a damaged left ventricle ranges from 15-20 mmHg.[7,14] This discrepancy reflects the ability of left atrial systole to boost the left ventricular end-diastolic pressure without raising the mean wedge pressure.[15] This elegant physiology allows optimal left ventricular filling without raising the hydrostatic pressure to levels causing pulmonary congestion. This concept is discussed further in Chapter 7. Since there is considerable individual variation, it is best to determine the optimal wedge pressure for each patient.

The mean wedge pressure is a reliable measure of the hydrostatic pressure in the pulmonary capillaries and can be used to aid in the diagnosis and management of pulmonary edema. To a certain extent, the desire to increase left ventricular filling pressure competes with the need to maintain pulmonary hydrostatic pressure at physiologic levels. In a critically ill patient, the physician is charged with optimizing this delicate balance. In the absence of lung injury or hypoalbuminemia, the threshold for hydrostatic pulmonary edema occurs at a mean wedge pressure of approximately 24 mmHg.[16,17] With chronic heart failure, pulmonary edema may not appear until the mean wedge pressure exceeds 30 mmHg, because of increased lymphatic drainage of the lung.[16,17] In the presence of hypoproteinemia or lung injury, pulmonary edema can occur with a mean wedge pressure below 20-25 mmHg.[16-18]

A mean wedge pressure less than 20 mmHg does not exonerate the heart as the cause of pulmonary edema. First of all, treatment with diuretics or vasodilators may have lowered the wedge pressure before it is measured. Second, the cardiac event which led to the pulmonary edema may have resolved by the time the wedge pressure is measured. Conditions such as myocardial ischemia or mitral regurgitation are notoriously brief. Routine hourly recording of the mean wedge pressure by the nursing staff can easily overlook these events. The wedge pressure is a dynamic measurement which changes on a beat-to-beat basis. A 5-minute episode of painless myocardial ischemia can raise the mean wedge pressure from 15 mmHg to 40 mmHg and result in radiographic pulmonary edema.[19] Although cardiogenic pulmonary edema may appear within minutes, its resolution requires hours to days. This results in the well-known lag between improvement in the wedge pressure and the chest x-ray.[17,20] It is unfortunate that the wedge pressure cannot be recorded continuously but prolonged inflation of the balloon would injure the pulmonary artery. Alternatively, the pulmonary artery pressure can be recorded continuously and the pulmonary artery diastolic pressure used to estimate the wedge pressure. Most modern bedside monitoring systems store hemodynamic data at 1 minute intervals for 24 hours or more providing a much better assessment of the dynamic nature of intracardiac pressure *(see Chapter 9)*.[20]

Confusion sometimes exists regarding interpretation of the mean wedge pressure in the presence of a large V wave. A large V wave raises the mean wedge pressure and contributes to the hydrostatic pressure in the pulmonary capillaries and the formation of pulmonary edema. In the presence of a large V wave, the mean wedge pressure remains a valid measure of the hydrostatic force prompting pulmonary edema formation. At the same time, a large V wave causes the mean wedge pressure to overestimate the left ventricular end-diastolic pressure. This is further discussed in Chapter 5.

Problems With The Wedge Pressure Measurement

The wedge pressure measurement is vulnerable to interpretation errors. Problems with wedge pressure interpretation can be divided into 2 general categories:[21]

- Cardiac conditions where the wedge pressure remains a valid measure of the left atrial pressure but is not a valid measure of the left ventricular end-diastolic pressure.

- Conditions where the wedge pressure is not a reliable measure of the left atrial pressure.

The mean wedge pressure is not an accurate measure of the left ventricular end-diastolic pressure in the following cardiac conditions:[12, 21]

- Mitral Stenosis: The mean wedge pressure overestimates the left ventricular filling pressure.

- Mitral regurgitation with a large V wave: The mean wedge pressure overestimates the left ventricular end-diastolic pressure. This is discussed further in Chapter 5.

- Noncompliant left ventricle (for example, with acute myocardial infarction): The mean wedge pressure underestimates the left ventricular end-diastolic pressure. This is discussed further in Chapter 7.

The use of the wedge pressure as an indirect measure of the left atrial pressure requires a direct blood filled vascular connection between the catheter tip and the left atrium. Any obstruction of this vascular window "disconnects" the wedge pressure measurement from the left atrial pressure measurement.

The location of the catheter tip becomes important because pulmonary capillary blood flow is not evenly distributed in the lungs.[22] Blood flow is greatest in the dependent areas of the lung and wedge pressure reflects true left atrial pressure when the catheter tip is in this zone.[22,23] Fortunately, in the supine patient, most pulmonary artery catheters will be directed to this area automatically by the blood flow itself. This concept is discussed in detail in Chapter 2. Based on these premises, the wedge pressure does not reflect the left atrial pressure in the following conditions.

- Abnormal pulmonary vascular bed (for example, with lung disease or pulmonary embolism).
- Elevated intrathoracic pressure causing collapse of the pulmonary capillary bed.
- A low mean left atrial pressure resulting in collapse of the flaccid pulmonary capillaries by a normal intrathoracic pressure.
- Location of the catheter tip within a poorly perfused segment of the lung.

It is easy to establish whether the wedge pressure recording is a reliable measure of the left atrial pressure. First, the presence of discrete A and V waves in the wedge tracing is direct evidence that a vascular communication between the catheter tip and the left atrium exists *(Figure 1.6)*. Second, the mean wedge pressure should always be less than the mean pulmonary artery pressure, otherwise blood flow would reverse.

Right Ventricular Pressure

Normal right ventricular pressures are:[1]

Systolic	15-30 mmHg
End-diastolic	2-8 mmHg

Right ventricular pressure is measured during insertion of the pulmonary artery catheter *(Figure 1.13)*. Most pulmonary artery

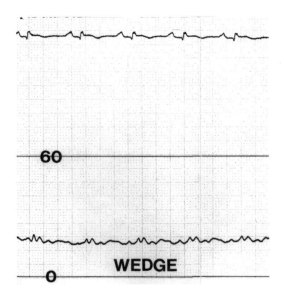

Figure 1.6 Wedge pressure waveform demonstrates only coarse oscillations rather than discrete A and V waves. The alveolar pressure is likely greater than the left atrial pressure preventing retrograde transmission of the A and V waves. The mean wedge pressure (end-expiration) is 16 mmHg but is likely an overestimate of the true left atrial pressure.
Scale = 0-60 mmHg;
Paper speed = 25 mm/sec.

catheters do not have a dedicated lumen for monitoring the right ventricular pressure. The mean right atrial pressure can be used to estimate the right ventricular end-diastolic pressure. The pulmonary artery systolic pressure can be used to estimate the right ventricular systolic pressure. It is therefore not necessary to directly measure the right ventricular pressure continuously.

Right Atrial Pressure

The normal right atrial pressure is 2-8 mmHg.[1] The right atrial pressure is governed by the right atrial blood volume, the right atrial compliance, the tricuspid valve function, and the right ventricular compliance. Interaction with the left atrium is mediated by the atrial septum and the pericardium. The mean right atrial pressure is composed of a series of positive and negative waveforms *(Figure 1.7)*.[24-26] These waveforms provide valuable clinical information. Two major positive pressure waves, the A wave and the V wave occur with each cardiac cycle. A third minor positive wave, the C wave can sometimes be recorded

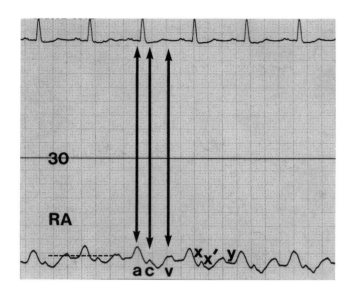

Figure 1.7 Normal right atrial pressure waveform. The rhythm is sinus. The mean right atrial pressure is 6 mmHg. The A wave (**a**) is the dominant positive pressure wave. The peak of the right atrial A wave follows the peak of the electrocardiographic P wave by about 80 msec. The right atrial C wave (**c**) occurs immediately following the QRS complex. The right atrial V wave (**v**) occurs on the downslope of the electrocardiographic T wave. The X (**x**) and Y (**y**) descents are similar in amplitude. Note that the C-wave interrupts the X descent yielding an X and X' (**x'**) descent. Scale = 0-30 mmHg; Paper speed = 25 mm/sec.

using bedside monitoring equipment. The A wave is due to atrial systole and is normally the dominant positive wave in the right atrial waveform *(Figure 1.7)*.[1] The A wave is accentuated when the filling of a noncompliant right ventricle requires a more forceful atrial systole. The peak of the right atrial A wave follows the peak of the electrocardiographic P wave by about 80 msec *(Figure 1.7)*. This time represents the intrinsic electromechanical delay inherent with all cardiac events plus the time required for the A wave to travel from the right atrium through the fluid-filled catheter system to the pressure transducer. This delay will vary slightly from patient to patient and from hospital to hospital.

The C wave is caused by the closure of the tricuspid valve at the onset of right ventricular systole. The C wave is a minor pressure wave but it can be recorded in the right atrial pressure waveform in most patients. The C wave immediately follows the QRS complex and follows the A wave by a time interval equal to the electrocardiographic P-R interval *(Figure 1.7)*. Prolongation of the P-R interval often makes the C wave more readily visible in the pressure waveform. The C wave marks the onset of right ventricular systole.

The V wave represents venous filling of the right atrium when ventricular systole has closed the tricuspid valve. The peak of the V wave occurs at the end of right ventricular systole and occurs within the electrocardiographic T wave *(Figure 1.7)*. The V wave is accentuated with conditions causing right atrial volume overload such as tricuspid regurgitation.

Two negative pressure deflections, the X and the Y descents follow the A and V waves respectively *(Figure 1.7)*. The X descent represents right atrial relaxation combined with the sudden downward motion of the atrioventricular junction during early right ventricular systole. Tricuspid regurgitation can attenuate or obliterate the X descent. The C wave, when visible, interrupts the X descent. When a C wave is visible, the initial descent is normal X and the final descent is named X' *(Figure 1.7)*.[26] The Y descent is caused by the rapid exit of blood from the right atrium into the right ventricle at the moment of tricuspid valve opening. The Y descent marks the onset of right ventricular diastole. Coincident with the X and Y descents, there is a surge of venous return to the right atrium from the superior and inferior vena cavae.

During inspiration, the mean right atrial pressure drops slightly and the positive A and V waves and negative X and Y descents are accentuated *(Figure 1.8)*.[27] Intuitively, one might expect the mean right atrial pressure to increase during inspiration because of augmented venous return to the right heart. As noted earlier, the measurement of intracardiac pressure

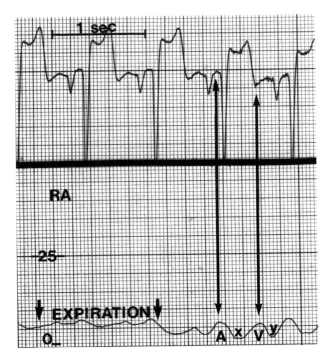

Figure 1.8 Influence of inspiration on the normal right atrial pressure waveform. The rhythm is sinus. The mean right atrial pressure (**RA**) is 6 mmHg at end-expiration. With inspiration, the mean right atrial pressure declines 2-3 mmHg. Note that the **A** and **V** waves and the X (**x**) and Y (**y**) descents are accentuated on inspiration. Scale = 0-25 mmHg; Paper speed = 25 mm/sec.

includes intrathoracic pressure *(Figure 1.9)*. With inspiration, the intrathoracic pressure declines overcoming the pressure augmentation of the increased venous return to the highly compliant right atrium. When the right atrium or right atrial pericardium is diseased and noncompliant, inspiration can cause an increase in the right atrial pressure (Kussmaul's sign).[6]

Clinical Use of the Right Atrial Pressure Measurement

The mean right atrial pressure is used clinically in the following ways:

- To assess the adequacy of right ventricular filling volume.
- To determine the hydrostatic pressure in the systemic veins.

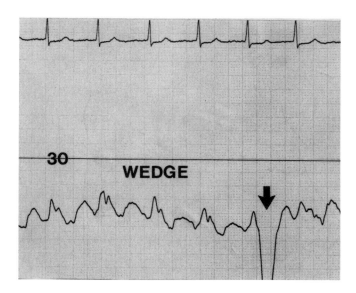

Figure 1.9 Effect of intrathoracic pressure change on the wedge pressure waveform. The patient has the hiccups. The sudden decrease in the intrathoracic pressure which occurs during the hiccup (**arrow**) is recorded by the pulmonary artery catheter. This influences the intracardiac pressure being measured. Scale = 0-30 mmHg; Paper speed = 25 mm/sec.

The mean right atrial pressure is a reliable measure of the right ventricular end-diastolic pressure if significant tricuspid stenosis or regurgitation is absent. In the normal heart, measurement of the right atrial pressure can be used to predict the left atrial pressure. For example, a low right atrial pressure predicts a low left atrial pressure and a high right atrial pressure predicts a high left atrial pressure. In the presence of cardiac disease, the right atrial pressure is a poor predictor of the left atrial pressure.[28] Significant cardiac disease mandates measurement of the wedge pressure to assess the left atrial pressure and the left ventricular filling pressure.[29,30]

The mean right atrial pressure provides a measure of the hydrostatic pressure in the systemic veins. This is an important variable in the formation of peripheral edema. Elevation of the right atrial pressure causes visceral congestion. It is not uncommon for a patient with decompensated heart failure to complain of abdominal pain because of hepatic and intestinal edema. An elevated right atrial pressure can promote pleural effusions since the lymphatic drainage of the lungs is into the jugular venous system via the thoracic duct.

The right atrial pressure waveform itself provides valuable clinical information. The pulmonary artery catheter has a dedicated lumen for monitoring the right atrial pressure. Right atrial pressure events can be directly recorded in fine detail *(Figure 1.7)*. Conditions such as pericardial tamponade, pericardial constriction, right ventricular infarction and tricuspid regurgitation can be suspected by careful analysis of the right atrial pressure waveform. The right atrial pressure waveform is equally valuable in the assessment of cardiac arrhythmias. All of these are discussed in detail in subsequent chapters. Finally, knowledge of the right atrial pressure relative to the wedge pressure is helpful. Elevation of the right atrial pressure out of proportion to the wedge pressure points to conditions such as pulmonary embolism and right ventricular infarction.

Arterial Pressure Waveforms

The hallmarks of an arterial pressure waveform are:[31]

- A wide pulse pressure (the pulse pressure equals the difference between the systolic pressure and the diastolic pressure).

- The presence of a dicrotic notch signifying closure of a semilunar valve.

The magnitude of the pulse pressure within the pulmonary artery or the aorta is in part due to the stroke volume ejected into that artery by the respective right or left ventricle. The pulse pressure therefore varies directly with the stroke volume. The pulse pressure measured within the pulmonary artery and aorta can be used in a general way to estimate the stroke volume of the right or left ventricles.[32]

Pulmonary Artery Pressure

Normal pulmonary artery pressures are:[1]

Systolic	15-30 mmHg
Diastolic	4-12 mmHg
Mean	9-18 mmHg

The normal pulmonary artery pulse pressure is approximately 15 mmHg *(Figure 1.5)*. The upstroke of the pulmonary artery pressure waveform reflects the onset of right ventricular ejection. The dicrotic notch is due to pulmonic valve closure and marks the end of right ventricular ejection. The peak of the pulmonary artery systolic pressure wave occurs within the electrocardiographic T wave *(Figure 1.5)*. Note that the peak pulmonary artery systolic pressure wave occurs earlier in time than the peak wedge pressure V wave *(Figure 1.5)*. As noted earlier, this observation is helpful when acute mitral regurgitation exists *(Chapter 5)*. In patients with normal pulmonary vascular resistance and no mitral valve obstruction, the pulmonary artery diastolic pressure is very close (2-4 mmHg) to both the mean wedge pressure and to the left ventricular end-diastolic pressure *(Figure 1.1)*.[33] In these patients, the pulmonary artery diastolic pressure can be substituted for the wedge pressure, thus minimizing the possibility of balloon injury to the pulmonary artery.[23]

When the pulmonary artery diastolic pressure exceeds the mean wedge pressure by ≥ 5 mmHg, conditions known to increase pulmonary vascular resistance (for example, pulmonary embolism) should be considered. The pulmonary artery diastolic pressure does not correlate well with the mean wedge pressure in the following situations:[34]

- Abnormal pulmonary vascular bed. The pulmonary artery diastolic pressure overestimates the mean wedge pressure.

- Mitral regurgitation with a large V wave. The pulmonary artery diastolic pressure underestimates the mean wedge pressure (see Chapter 5).

Aortic Pressure

Normal arterial pressures are:[1]

Systolic	100-140 mmHg
Diastolic	60-90 mmHg
Mean	70-105 mmHg

The normal aortic pulse pressure is 40-50 mmHg *(Figure 1.10)*. The upstroke of the aortic pressure wave reflects the onset of left ventricular ejection. The aortic systolic pressure equals the left ventricular systolic pressure in the absence of left ventricular outflow obstruction (for example with aortic stenosis). With inspiration, the normal arterial systolic pressure declines by 5-10 mmHg *(Figure 1.10)*.[27] The dicrotic notch is due to aortic valve closure and marks the end of left ventricular ejection *(Figure 1.10)*. The relation between the peak of the aortic systolic pressure and the electrocardiogram varies widely and is dependent on the location of the arterial pressure monitoring catheter with respect to the aortic valve. The arterial pressure waveform itself changes with the location of the catheter. As the pressure monitoring lumen is moved from the central aorta to a peripheral artery, the systolic pressure increases while the diastolic and mean pressures decrease.[6,23] The dicrotic notch occurs later and at a lower arterial pressure.[6,23] In the presence of profound arterial vasoconstriction (as for example with shock), the peripheral arterial systolic pressure can be significantly lower than the central aortic pressure.[6,23] Obviously, the patient's clinical state should dictate the anatomic site selected for pressure monitoring.

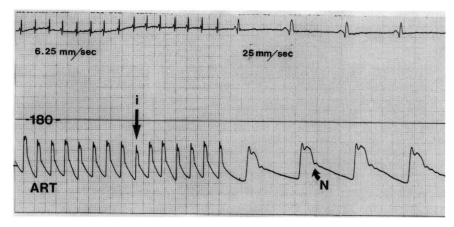

Figure 1.10 Normal arterial (**ART**) pressure waveform recorded from the femoral artery. The arterial pressure is 140/90 mmHg. At left, a slow paper speed (6.25 mm/sec) illustrates the normal influence of inspiration (**i**) on the arterial pressure. In this patient, inspiration causes a 6 mmHg decrease in the systolic arterial pressure. At right, a paper speed of 25 mm/sec illustrates the normal features of an arterial pressure wave. These include a prominent pulse pressure (50 mmHg in this patient) and a dicrotic notch (**N**) signifying closure of the aortic valve. The crisp dicrotic notch indicates a properly responsive catheter system. Scale = 0-180 mmHg.

The Pulmonary Artery Catheter[35-37]

The standard pulmonary artery catheter is radiopaque, 110 cm long, and has black distance marking rings at 10 cm intervals. The "working anatomy" of the pulmonary artery catheter is shown in Figure 1.11. The proximal lumen of the pulmonary artery catheter is located 30 cm from the catheter tip and in most patients will lie within the right atrium. Right atrial pressure events are recorded directly through this lumen. Cold solution can be injected through this lumen to perform the thermodilution cardiac output. In addition, right atrial oxygen saturation can be measured by obtaining a blood sample from the proximal lumen. The distal lumen is located at the catheter

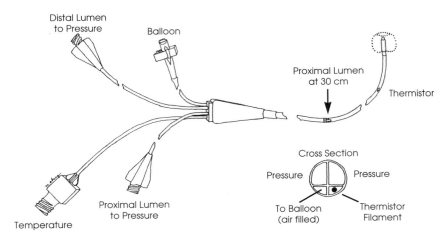

Figure 1.11 Diagram depicting the working anatomy of the pulmonary artery catheter. Two pressure monitoring lumens are present. A proximal lumen at 30 cm allows right atrial pressure measurement. This lumen is also used for injection of cold solution to perform the thermodilution cardiac output. A distal lumen at the catheter tip allows pulmonary artery and wedge pressure measurement. A thermistor near the catheter tip measures pulmonary artery blood temperature and is used for thermodilution cardiac output measurement. A balloon at the tip can be inflated with room air to measure wedge pressure. cm = centimeters. Courtesy: NB Aberg.

tip and allows the direct measurement of the pulmonary artery pressure. Inflation of the balloon occludes that pulmonary artery segment and yields an indirect measurement of the left atrial pressure (the wedge pressure).

Pulmonary artery oxygen saturation can be measured continuously through the catheter tip with the addition of a fiberoptic bundle. A thermistor located 4 cm from the catheter tip measures the pulmonary artery blood temperature (the ultimate core temperature) and is used for the thermodilution cardiac output measurement. The following physiologic data are thus readily available using bedside monitoring techniques: heart rate, aortic pressure, pulmonary artery pressure, pulmonary capillary wedge pressure, right atrial pressure, pulmonary artery oxygen saturation, thermodilution cardiac output, and pulmonary artery blood temperature.

Bedside Pressure Measurement Technique[23,37]

The standard equipment used for recording bedside intracardiac pressures is shown in Figure 1.12. The pulmonary artery catheter is fluid-filled and connected to a pressure transducer via noncompliant pressure tubing. For optimal recordings, the length of this tubing should not exceed 3-4 feet and the number of stopcocks kept to a minimum. A two-channel physiologic recorder is essential because intracardiac pressure waveforms cannot be properly interpreted without a simultaneously recorded single-lead electrocardiogram. The equipment used to measure intracardiac pressures includes a transducer, an amplifier, and an oscilloscope. Intracardiac pressure events are transmitted from the heart and great vessels through the fluid filled catheter to a transducer. The transducer *(Figure 1.12)* converts mechanical events into electrical signals. The transducer is fluid filled and contains a thin diaphragm which moves in response to cardiac pressure events. The motion of the diaphragm generates an electrical signal which is then amplified and displayed at the bedside on an oscilloscope. The magnitude of the electrical signal is proportional to the displacement of the diaphragm. Prior to measurement of intracardiac pressures, the transducer must be both zeroed and calibrated.

Zeroing and Calibrating the Transducer[37,38]

Intracardiac pressures are measured relative to atmospheric pressure. The atmospheric pressure is assigned a value of zero. The transducer is equipped with a stopcock to allow establishing the zero pressure reference. The air-fluid interface in this stopcock is the zero reference point *(Figure 1.12)*. This zero reference point must be level with the heart. The heart is assumed to be at the mid-chest, halfway between the anterior and posterior chest walls *(Figure 1.12)*. This point is marked with an indelible marker for future reference. Each time pressures are measured, the patient should be positioned with the heart at the level of the zero reference point.

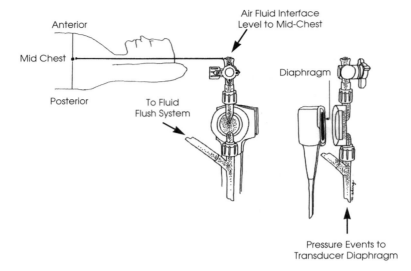

Figure 1.12 Pressure transducer (front and side views) and its relation to the patient. Pressure events from the patient's heart are transmitted to the fluid filled transducer dome causing the diaphragm to move. Motion of the diaphragm generates an electrical current proportional to the magnitude of the pressure events. This electrical current is amplified and displayed on an oscilloscope at the bedside. The zero reference point is the air fluid interface at the stopcock on top of the transducer. This should be level with the patient's mid-chest (heart). Courtesy: NB Aberg.

The calibration procedure insures that each mmHg of pressure is converted to a proportional electrical signal. This allows precise measurement of the intracardiac pressures. The calibration technique is usually performed electronically at the bedside.

Catheter Insertion[36,37]

Prior to catheter insertion, the transducer must be zeroed and calibrated. It is wise to check the response of the system to mechanical events before inserting the catheter. This can be performed using the fast flush technique[36,38,39] *(Figure 1.13)*. During insertion, pressure is monitored through the distal catheter lumen. The pulmonary artery catheter can usually be inserted without fluoroscopy because each cardiac chamber has a characteristic pressure waveform. Familiarity with these waveforms allows the operator to guide the catheter from the right atrium to the right ventricle, pulmonary artery, and wedge position while watching the oscilloscope (*Figure 1.13*). The distance markers on the catheter are also helpful.[37] If insertion is performed from the internal jugular or subclavian veins the superior vena cava is reached at about 10-15 cm. The balloon can be safely inflated at this point provided that a pressure waveform is visible on the oscilloscope and the waveform demonstrates respiratory variation (confirming an intrathoracic location). In general, the right atrium is reached at 15-20 cm, the right ventricle at 30-40 cm, the pulmonary artery at 45-55 cm and the wedge at 45-60 cm.[37] If greater distances are encountered then the catheter is likely coiling in the right atrium or right ventricle. After insertion, proper catheter position should be confirmed with a chest x-ray.

Pressure Waveform Analysis

The interpretation of pressure waveform data requires a solid understanding of the normal sequence of events of the cardiac cycle.[6,11,26] Before analyzing the pressure waveforms, the physician must assess the cardiac rhythm since the cardiac electrical activity governs all mechanical events. The following steps are recommended for proper pressure data analysis:

- Check that the pressure transducer has been properly zeroed to the estimated level of the heart.

- Check the dynamic pressure response of the system using the fast-flush test[39] alternatively, a crisp dicrotic notch on the pulmonary artery tracing indicates a properly responsive system.

- Choose the pressure scale which best accommodates the intracardiac pressure being measured.

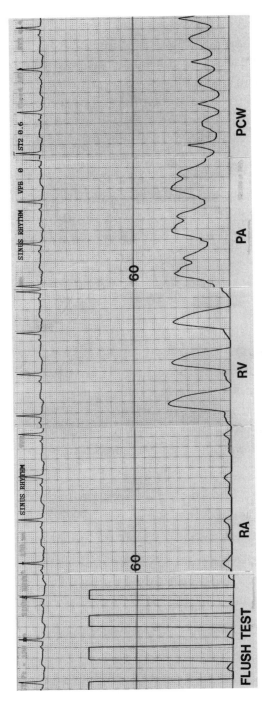

Figure 1.13 Pressure recordings obtained during bedside insertion of a pulmonary artery catheter. At left, a "flush test" confirms proper operation of the equipment before insertion. Each cardiac chamber has a signature pressure waveform which allows the operator to know the location of the distal lumen as it is advanced through the heart into proper position. Notice that the right atrial (**RA**) pressure is equal to the right ventricular (**RV**) diastolic pressure. The RV systolic pressure equals the pulmonary artery (**PA**) systolic pressure. The PA diastolic pressure equals the mean wedge (**PCW**) pressure. As the catheter moves from the RV to the PA, the diastolic pressure suddenly increases and a dicrotic notch appears. As the catheter moves from PA to wedge, the mean pressure suddenly drops with appearance of A and V waves. Scale = 0-60 mmHg; Paper speed = 25 mm/sec.

- Choose an electrocardiographic lead which best illustrates atrial activity.

- Record the single-lead electrocardiogram together with the pressure waveform at a paper speed of 25 mm/sec.

- Include 2-4 respiratory cycles and measure the intracardiac pressure at end-expiration.[6]

- Identify the A wave and the V wave in the right atrial and the wedge pressure waveforms by drawing a vertical line from the positive pressure waves to the electrocardiogram.

- Identify the X descent and the Y descent.

- Assess the effect of spontaneous inspiration on the mean right atrial pressure.

- If indicated, perform the hepatojugular reflux test while recording the right atrial pressure.[40]

- Identify the systolic pressure and the diastolic pressure in the pulmonary artery and aortic pressure waveforms and measure the respective pulse pressures; identify the dicrotic notch on each arterial pressure waveform.

- Measure the pressure gradient between the pulmonary artery diastolic pressure and the mean wedge pressure. This should be ≤ 5 mmHg.[23,34]

- Measure the ratio of the mean right atrial pressure/mean wedge pressure. Normally, this is approximately 0.5.

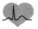 **Key Points: Normal Physiology**

- The mean right atrial pressure is a measure of both the hydrostatic pressure in the systemic veins and the right ventricular end-diastolic (filling) pressure.

- The wedge pressure is an indirect measurement of the left atrial pressure. The mean left atrial pressure is a valuable estimate of both the hydrostatic pressure in the lungs and the left ventricular end-diastolic (filling) pressure.

- The wedge pressure is a valid measure of the left atrial pressure when discrete A and V waves are present in the wedge pressure waveform. This signifies retrograde transmission of left atrial events to the catheter tip.

- The wedge pressure is not a valid measure of the left atrial pressure when intrathoracic pressure exceeds the distending pressure of the pulmonary capillary bed. Parenchymal lung disease, volume depletion, pulmonary vascular disease and catheter tip malposition are common causes. In these conditions, the wedge pressure is more a measure of intrathoracic pressure than transmural left atrial pressure.

- The mean wedge pressure underestimates the left ventricular end-diastolic pressure in the presence of a noncompliant left ventricle.

- The mean wedge pressure overestimates the left ventricular end-diastolic pressure in the presence of a large V wave. Nonetheless, this V wave contributes to the hydrostatic pressure in the pulmonary capillary bed.

- The pulmonary artery diastolic pressure is normally a close estimate of both the mean wedge pressure and the left ventricular end-diastolic pressure. An increase in the pulmonary vascular resistance disrupts this relationship.

- The pulmonary artery diastolic pressure underestimates the mean wedge pressure in the presence of a large V wave.

Chapter 1 References

1. Grossman W, Barry WH. Cardiac catheterization. In: Braunwald E, ed. *Heart Disease: A Textbook of Cardiovascular Medicine.* Philadelphia: WB Saunders, 1988;247-252.

2. Shabetai R. *The Pericardium.* New York: Grune & Stratton, 1981;66-67.

3. Braunwald E, Frahm CJ. Studies on Starling's Law of the heart observations on the hemodynamic function of the left atrium in man. *Circulation* 1961;24:633-642.

4. Braunwald E, Ross J, Jr. The ventricular end-diastolic pressure. *Am J Med* 1963;34:147-150.

5. Parker JO, Case RB. Normal left ventricular function. *Circulation* 1979;60:4-12.

6. Schlant RC, Sonnenblick EH. Normal physiology of the cardiovascular system. In: Hurst JW, ed. *The Heart: Arteries and Veins.* New York: McGraw-Hill, 1986; Plates 1 & 2;51-72.

7. Crexells C, Chatterjee K, Forrester JS. Optimal level of filling pressure in the left side of the heart in acute myocardial infarction. *N Engl J Med* 1973;289:1263-1266.

8. Luchsinger PC, Seipp HW, Patel DJ. Relationship of pulmonary artery wedge pressure to left atrial pressure in man. *Circ Res* 1962;11:315-318.

9. Connally DC, Kirklin JW, Wood EH. The relationship between pulmonary artery wedge pressure and left atrial pressure in man. *Circ Res* 1954;2:434-440.

10. Shaffer AB, Silber EN. Factors influencing the character of the pulmonary arterial wedge pressure. *Am Heart J* 1956;51:522-532.

11. Braunwald E, Fishman AP, Cournand A. Time relationship of dynamic events in the cardiac chambers, pulmonary artery, and aorta in man. *Circ Res* 1956;4:100-107.

12. O'Quinn R, Marini JJ. Pulmonary artery occlusion pressure: Clinical physiology, measurement and interpretation. *Am Rev Respir Dis.* 1983;128:319-326.

13. Sapru RP, Taylor SH, Donald KW. Comparison of the pulmonary wedge pressure with the left ventricular end-diastolic pressure in man. *Clin Sci* 1968;34:125-140.

14. Russell RO, Rackley CE, Pombo J, Hunt D, Potanin C, Dodge HT. Effects of increasing left ventricular filling pressure in patients with acute myocardial infarction. *J Clin Invest* 1970;49:1539-1550.

15. Rahimtoola SH, Ehsani A, Sinno MZ. Left atrial transport function in myocardial infarction. Importance of its booster pump function. *Am J Med* 1975;59:686-694.

16. Sprung CL, Rackow EC, Fein IA, Jacob AI, Isikoff SK. The spectrum of pulmonary edema. Differentiation of cardiogenic, intermediate, and noncardiogenic forms of pulmonary edema. *Am Rev Respir Dis* 1981;124:718-722.

17. McHugh TJ, Forrester JS, Adler L, Zion D, Swan HJC. Pulmonary vascular congestion in acute myocardial infarction: hemodynamics and radiologic correlations. *Ann Intern Med* 1972;76:29-33.

18. Guyton AC, Lindsay AW. Effect of elevated left atrial pressure and decreased plasma protein concentration on the development of pulmonary edema. *Circ Res* 1959;7:649-657.

19. Sharkey SW, Aberg NB. Hemodynamic evidence of painless myocardial ischemia with acute pulmonary edema in coronary disease. *Am Heart J* 1995;129:188-91.

20. McHugh TJ, Adler L, Zion D, Swan HJC, Forrester JS. Simultaneous hemodynamic radiologic and physiologic evaluation of left ventricle failure in acute myocardial infarction. *Chest* 1970;58:285-289.

21. Tumen KJ, Carrol GC, Ivankovich AD. Pitfalls in interpretation of pulmonary artery catheter data. *J Cardiothor Anesth* 1989;3:625-641.

22. West JB, Dollery CT, Naimark A. Distribution of pulmonary blood flow in isolated lung: relation to vascular and alveolar pressures. *J Appl Physiol* 1964;19:713-724.

23. Amin DK, Shah PK, Swan HJC. The Swan-Ganz Catheter: Tips on interpreting results. *J Crit Illness* 1986;1:40-48.

24. MacKenzie J. The interpretation of the pulsations in the jugular veins. *Am J Med Sci* 1907;134:12-34.

25. Mackay IFS. The true venous pulse wave, central and peripheral. *Am Heart J* 1967;74:48-57.

26. Constant J. The X prime descent in jugular contour nomenclature and recognition. *Am Heart J* 1974;88:372-379.

27. Lauson HD, Bloomfield RA, Cournand A. The influence of the respiration in the circulation in man. *Am J Med* 1946;1:315-336.

28. Bell H, Stubbs D, Pugh D. Reliability of central venous pressure as an indicator of left atrial pressure: A study in patients with mitral valve disease. *Chest* 1971;59:169-173.

29. Mangano DT. Monitoring pulmonary arterial pressure in coronary artery disease. *Anesthesiology* 1980;53:364-370.

30. Forrester JS, Diamond G, McHugh TH, Swan HJC. Filling pressures in the right and left sides of the heart in acute myocardial infarction. *N Engl J Med* 1971;285:190-193.

31. O'Rourke MF. The arterial pulse in health and disease. *Am Heart J* 1971;82:687-702.

32. Starr I. Clinical tests of the simple method of estimating cardiac stroke volume from blood pressure and age. *Circulation* 1954;9:664-681.

33. Jenkins BS, Bradley RD, Branthwaite MA. Evaluation of pulmonary arterial end-diastolic pressure as an indirect estimate of left atrial mean pressure. *Circulation* 1970;42:75-78.

34. Levin RI, Glissman E. Left atrial pulmonary artery wedge pressure relation: Effect of elevated pulmonary vascular resistance. *Am J Cardiol* 1985;55:856-857.

35. Swan HJC, Ganz W, Forrester J, Marcus H, Diamond G, Chonette D. Catheterization of the heart in man with use of a flow-directed balloon-tipped catheter. *N Engl J Med* 1970;283:447-451.

36. Civetta JMO. Pulmonary artery catheter insertion. In: Sprung CL, ed. *The Pulmonary Artery Catheter.* Baltimore: University Park Press, 1983;37.

37. Amin DK, Shah PK, Swan HJC. The technique of inserting a Swan-Ganz Catheter. *J Crit Illness* 1986;1:1147-1156.

38. Kett DH, Schein RMH. Techniques for pulmonary artery catheter insertion. In: Sprung CL, ed. *The Pulmonary Artery Catheter.* Closter: Critical Care Research Associates Inc., 1993;43-45.

39. Gardner RM. Direct blood pressure measurement. Dynamic response requirements. *Anesthesiology* 1981;54:227-236.

40. Sochowski RA, Dubbin JD, Naqvi SZ. Clinical and hemodynamic assessment of the hepatojugular reflux. *Am J Cardiol* 1990;66:1002-1006.

CHAPTER 2

RESPIRATION

Human anatomy dictates that the heart resides within the thorax. Consequently, the act of breathing influences the heart and hemodynamic measurements.[1] Respiration impacts hemodynamic measurements in several ways.

Intrathoracic pressure is transmitted directly to the heart; all bedside intracardiac pressure measurements represent the sum of intracardiac pressure plus intrathoracic pressure. The transmural intracardiac pressure is a measure of the distending pressure or preload. The transmural pressure is equal to the intracardiac pressure measurement minus the intrathoracic pressure measurement *(Figure 2.1)*. In practice, the transmural pressure is rarely determined because measurement of the intrathoracic pressure is too difficult. In the absence of lung disease, the intrathoracic pressure at end-expiration approaches zero.[2] Bedside intracardiac pressure measurements therefore should be determined at end-expiration to minimize the effects of intrathoracic pressure.[2] In the presence of significant lung disease, the intrathoracic pressure is often well above zero which can lead to a serious overestimate of the transmural intracardiac pressure *(Figure 2.2)*.

The wedge pressure measurement is particularly sensitive to the intrathoracic pressure. For the wedge pressure to accurately reflect the left atrial pressure, a blood filled connection between

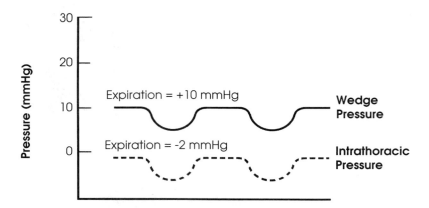

Figure 2.1 Schematic depicting the relation of measured wedge pressure to intrathoracic pressure in a normal person. At end-expiration, the measured wedge pressure is 10 mmHg and the intrathoracic pressure -2 mmHg. The transmural wedge pressure is therefore 10 - (-2) mmHg = 12 mmHg. The transmural wedge pressure is very close to the measured wedge pressure because the end-expiratory intrathoracic pressure is nearly atmospheric.

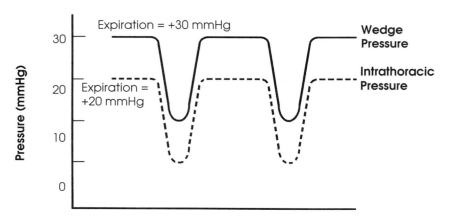

Figure 2.2 Schematic depicting the relation of measured wedge pressure to intrathoracic pressure in a person with severe lung disease. There is a 20 mmHg swing in the intrathoracic pressure between inspiration and expiration. At end-expiration, the measured wedge pressure is 30 mmHg and the intrathoracic pressure is 20 mmHg. The transmural wedge pressure is therefore 30 - (20) mmHg = 10 mmHg. The measured wedge pressure seriously overestimates the transmural wedge pressure because of the high level of intrathoracic pressure.

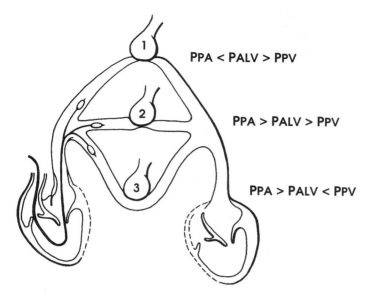

PPA < PALV > PPV

PPA > PALV > PPV

PPA > PALV < PPV

Figure 2.3 Physiologic lung zones and their relation to the pulmonary artery catheter. In Zones 1 and 2, the alveolar pressure (**PALV**) exceeds the pulmonary venous pressure (**PPV**) preventing retrograde transmission of left atrial events when the catheter is wedged. In Zone 3, the pulmonary venous pressure exceeds alveolar pressure allowing retrograde transmission of the left atrial A and V waves when the catheter is wedged. Gravity has an important effect on these zones. In the upright position, Zone 3 is located inferiorly. In the supine position, Zone 3 is located posteriorly. PPA = pulmonary artery pressure. Adapted from Marini JJ et al. *Am Rev Respir Dis.* 1983;128:319-326.

the catheter tip and the left atrium must be present.[3]   When this prerequisite is satisfied. retrograde transmission of left atrial mechanical events occur through the pulmonary capillary bed. For a patent blood filled column to exist, the tip of the pulmonary artery catheter must be located in a lung segment where the pulmonary venous pressure exceeds the alveolar pressure *(Figure 2.3)*. Based on the relation between pulmonary vascular and alveolar pressures, three physiologic zones exist in the lung *(Figure 2.3)*.[3,4]

The physiologic lung zones are as follows:[4]

Zone 1 = Alveolar pressure > both pulmonary artery and
pulmonary venous pressures

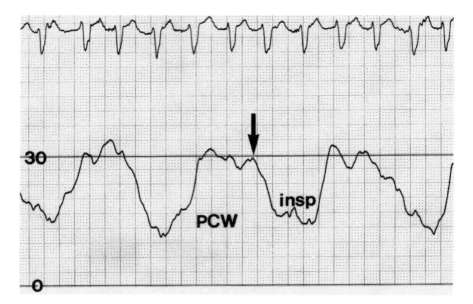

Figure 2.4 Influence of labored respiration on the wedge pressure waveform (**PCW**). With inspiration (**insp**) the wedge pressure drops abruptly. The respiratory excursion (difference between expiration and inspiration) exceeds 15 mmHg. The A and V waves are absent from the pressure waveform because alveolar pressure exceeds pulmonary capillary pressure. The end-expiratory wedge pressure (**arrow**) is 30 mmHg. This measurement is a significant overestimate of the transmural left atrial pressure in this patient with bilateral pneumonia.
Scale = 0-30 mmHg; Paper speed = 25 mm/sec.

Zone 2 = Pulmonary artery pressure > alveolar pressure > pulmonary venous pressure

Zone 3 = Pulmonary artery and pulmonary venous pressures > alveolar pressure

Fortunately, most of the lung is in Zone 3 in the supine patient and the balloon tipped pulmonary artery catheter is naturally directed to this zone because pulmonary blood flow is directed to Zone 3.[3] The presence of distinct A and V waves on the wedge pressure waveform indicates the catheter tip is in a Zone 3 lung segment. Whenever the alveolar pressure exceeds the pulmonary venous pressure (Zones 1 & 2), the A and V waves disappear from the wedge pressure waveform *(Figure 2.4)*. In this situation, the wedge pressure becomes a measurement of the alveolar pressure rather than the left atrial pressure. Zone 1 or 2 conditions can be created by hypovolemia or by conditions which elevate the alveolar pressure (severe lung disease or positive pressure ventilation - *Figure 2.5*).[2-7] In some patients, it is not possible or practical to achieve a Zone 3 location for the catheter.

Intrathoracic pressure also has indirect effects on the heart.[1-8] An increase in the intrathoracic pressure reduces venous return to the right and left atria whereas a decrease in the intrathoracic pressure promotes venous return to the atria.[1] At the same time, an increase in the intrathoracic pressure reduces the impedance to the left ventricular ejection (the higher the intrathoracic pressure, the easier it is for the left ventricle to eject blood out of the thorax).

The decrease in the intrathoracic pressure which occurs during normal inspiration translates into an increase in the impedance to left ventricular ejection. With a normal left ventricle, this effect is barely noticeable. However, when left ventricular stroke volume is reduced, inspiration can have a significant effect on the stroke volume and consequently the blood pressure. For example, it is possible to observe a striking inspiratory fall in the blood pressure (pulsus paradoxus) in patients with hypovolemic shock.[9] This is due primarily to the effect of intrathoracic pressure on impedance to ejection.

Normal Respiration

The normal end-expiratory intrathoracic pressure is -3 to -4 mmHg which drops to -7 to -8 mmHg at end-inspiration.[10] Inspiration is an active process which requires the contraction of the diaphragm and the external intercostal muscles.[11] Expiration is passive during quiet breathing in normal individuals.[11] The influence of the intrathoracic pressure on the intracardiac pressure measurement is least at end-expiration. For this reason, intracardiac pressure measurements are usually recorded at end-expiration when intrathoracic pressure is near zero.[1]

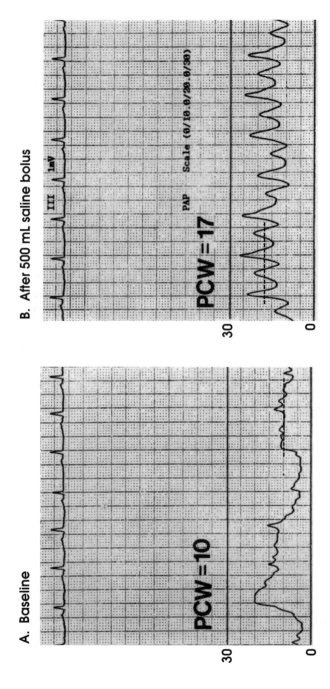

Figure 2.5   Effect of volume status on the wedge pressure waveform.   **Panel A:**   The end-expiratory wedge pressure is 10 mmHg, but distinct A and V waves are not present.   This indicates that alveolar pressure exceeds pulmonary capillary pressure (Zone 1 or 2 condition).   The wedge pressure measurement therefore overestimates the transmural left atrial pressure.   **Panel B:**   The wedge-pressure recording was repeated after a 500 mL normal saline bolus.   The end-expiratory wedge pressure is now 17 mmHg.   The presence of distinct A and V waves indicates a Zone 3 condition.   The wedge pressure measurement is now an accurate reflection of the left atrial pressure. Scale = 0-30 mmHg; Paper speed = 25 mm/sec.

Activation of the inspiratory muscles decreases intrathoracic pressure. This in turn increases the venous return to the right atrium and, to a lesser extent, the left atrium.[1] Despite these inspiratory increases in cardiac filling, there is a seemingly paradoxic decrease in the right atrial, wedge, and pulmonary artery pressures *(Figure 2.6)*. This occurs because the inspiratory decrease in the intrathoracic pressure exceeds the inspiratory increase in the transmural intracardiac pressures. The left and right atria are normally very compliant structures. They accept the increased venous return with a minimal increase in transmural pressure. With myocardial or pericardial disease, atrial compliance diminishes and increased venous return causes a major increase in the transmural pressure. Under these conditions, Kussmaul's sign (an inspiratory increase in right atrial pressure) can be observed.

Labored Respiration

Patients with lung disease often have significant increases in the intrathoracic pressure. In these patients, the transmural intracardiac pressure measurements are "overwhelmed" by the intrathoracic pressure *(Figure 2.2)*. Patients with labored breathing have large excursions of intrathoracic pressure which are transmitted to the pulmonary artery catheter; the pressure tracing resembles a roller coaster ride *(Figure 2.4)*. Intrathoracic pressure at end-expiration is often markedly elevated causing a serious overestimation of the transmural intracardiac pressures.[2,3,11] When more than 10-15 mmHg of respiratory variation is seen in the wedge pressure tracing, the end-expiratory pressure wedge pressure measurement is likely to be a significant overestimate of the transmural left atrial pressure.[2,11,12] The ideal approach to this patient would be to measure the intrathoracic pressure directly and subtract if from the intracardiac pressure. This is usually not feasible. Efforts to encourage quiet breathing should be attempted but may be impossible. In some cases, pressure recording while the patient sips water through a straw may reduce

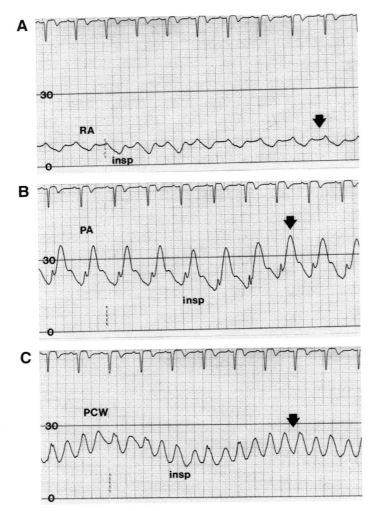

Figure 2.6 Effect of normal respiration on the intracardiac pressures. **Panel A:** The right atrial (**RA**) pressure drops slightly (1-2 mmHg) on inspiration (**insp**). **Panel B:** The pulmonary artery (**PA**) systolic and diastolic pressures fall (3-4 mmHg) on inspiration (**insp**). **Panel C:** The wedge pressure (**PCW**) declines (5-6 mmHg) on inspiration (**insp**). Despite the measured decrease in the cardiac pressures, the venous return and pulmonary artery flow increase with inspiration. The intracardiac pressures should be measured at end-expiration (**bold arrows**).
Scale = 0-30 mmHg; Paper speed = 25 mm/sec.

the intrathoracic pressure variation.[2] If the large intrathoracic pressure excursions persist, the following is recommended:

- Always measure the intracardiac pressure at end-expiration. This provides consistency.

- Accept the fact that the end-expiratory intrathoracic pressure in these patients is usually well above zero. The end-expiratory pressure measurement will thus be an overestimate of the transmural pressure.

- If the clinical situation demands precise knowledge of the transmural intracardiac pressure, then it is best to measure the mean intrathoracic pressure (or its surrogate, the intraesophageal pressure) and subtract this from the mean intracardiac pressure measurement.[13,14]

These recommendations can be applied to the measurement of the pulmonary artery, right atrial, and wedge pressures.

Mechanical Ventilation

Mechanical ventilators alter normal physiology. Intrathoracic pressure is increased and venous return is decreased during inspiration *(Figure 2.7)*. This is 180° of normal spontaneous inspiration. Even with mechanical ventilation, intrathoracic pressure is closest to atmospheric pressure at end-expiration and intracardiac pressures should be measured at this point.[3] Patients on mechanical ventilators often have serious lung disease and large excursions in the intrathoracic pressure may be present similar to those described in spontaneously breathing patients with respiratory distress. If large excursions of intrathoracic pressure are present (>10-15 mmHg), patients may be temporarily paralyzed and sedated to obtain a reliable measurement[2,15] *(Figure 2.8)*. With mechanical ventilation, it is common for alveolar pressure to exceed pulmonary venous pressure during inspiration (Zone 1 or 2 condition).[2,3] With expiration and the resulting drop in the intrathoracic pressure, Zone 3 conditions usually prevail.

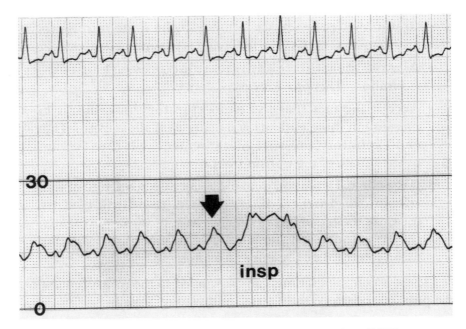

Figure 2.7 Effect of mechanical ventilation on the wedge (**PCW**) pressure measurement. On inspiration (**insp**), the wedge pressure increases 5 mmHg due to the positive intrathoracic pressure delivered by the ventilator. Despite the increase in the measured pressure, venous return actually decreases. The wedge pressure should be measured at end-expiration (**arrow**). Scale = 0-30 mmHg; Paper speed = 25 mm/sec.

Positive end-expiratory pressure (PEEP) further complicates the hemodynamic measurements of patients on ventilators.[3,16] PEEP can be deliberately applied through the ventilator or be the result of gas trapping and increased end-expiratory lung volumes ("AUTO-PEEP").[17] The result is transmission of this airway pressure to the heart. PEEP promotes alveolar pressures which exceed pulmonary venous pressure (Zone 1 and 2 conditions). In general, with PEEP levels below 10 cm H_2O (7 mmHg), the effect on bedside intracardiac pressure measurements is small. At levels above 10 cm H_2O, PEEP significantly influences the bedside pressure measurement[2] *(Figure 2.9)*. The degree to which PEEP is transmitted to the pleural space and heart varies with the individual.[2,18] Therefore, one cannot simply subtract the level of

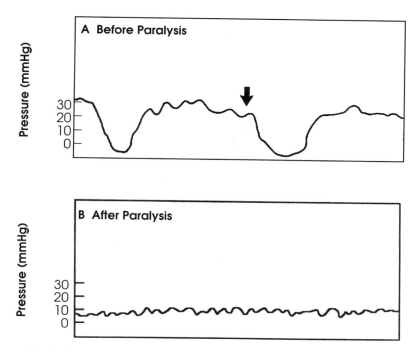

Figure 2.8 Schematic demonstrating the effect of respiratory distress on the end-expiration wedge pressure.

Panel A: Recording of wedge pressure from a patient on a mechanical ventilator with severe respiratory distress. There is marked respiratory fluctuation in the wedge pressure. The end-expiration wedge pressure (**arrow**) is 25 mmHg which is an overestimate of the transmural left atrial pressure.

Panel B: Repeat recording of the wedge pressure after paralysis. The respiratory fluctuation in the wedge pressure is now trivial. The end-expiratory wedge pressure is 8 mmHg with transmission of the A and V waves now present. This measurement is a much more accurate reflection of the left ventricular filling pressure. Adapted from Leatherman and Marini[7] with permission.

PEEP from the intracardiac pressure measurement. Even knowledge of the intrathoracic pressure itself may not help since the transmission of PEEP varies within the thorax.[18,19] Discontinuation of PEEP to make hemodynamic measurements is not advised.[2,20] First, the patient may become hypoxemic. This could lead to a change in cardiac function and an increase in

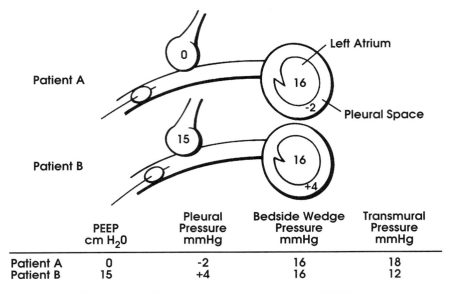

	PEEP cm H_2O	Pleural Pressure mmHg	Bedside Wedge Pressure mmHg	Transmural Pressure mmHg
Patient A	0	-2	16	18
Patient B	15	+4	16	12

Figure 2.9 Effect of positive end-expiratory pressure (**PEEP**) on transmural pressure. The baseline pleural pressure is assumed to be -2 mmHg for both patients A and B. The measured wedge pressure is identical (16 mmHg) for both patients. In patient A (without PEEP), the transmural cardiac pressure is: 16 mmHg - (-2 mmHg) = 18 mmHg. In patient B, 15 cm H_2O (12 mmHg) of PEEP is added, 50% of which (6 mmHg) is transmitted to the heart. This results in an increase in the pleural pressure from -2 mmHg to +4 mmHg. The transmural pressure in this patient is: 16 mmHg - (+4 mmHg) = 12 mmHg. Although the wedge pressures of the two patients are identical, the effective filling pressure of Patient A exceeds that of Patient B. Adapted from Leatherman and Marini[7] with permission.

pulmonary vascular resistance.[3] Second, sudden removal of PEEP changes the venous return to both sides of the heart creating an entirely new set of hemodynamic circumstances. In short, there is currently no practical solution to the problem which high PEEP levels impose on hemodynamic measurements. It is best to carefully assess the effects of therapy on the patient's clinical status. For example, if the patient is suffering from oliguria, a volume challenge can be given followed by assessment of its effect on the wedge pressure, the stroke volume, the oxygen saturation, and the urine flow.

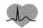 **Key Points: Respiration and Hemodynamic Measurements**

- Intrathoracic pressure is transmitted to the heart. All bedside pressure measurements reflect the sum of the transmural (distending) intracardiac pressure and the intrathoracic pressure. In normal individuals, the influence of intrathoracic pressure is minimal. In patients with lung disease, intrathoracic pressure may be very high and "overwhelm" the transmural intracardiac pressure. The wedge pressure is not an accurate measure of left ventricular filling volume in these patients.

- The wedge pressure measurement is particularly vulnerable to elevated intrathoracic pressure; a high intrathoracic pressure blocks retrograde transmission of left atrial pressure events to the catheter tip.

- Intrathoracic pressure influences cardiac venous return (preload) and left ventricular ejection (afterload). These effects indirectly alter hemodynamic measurements.

- Labored breathing (both on and off a ventilator) causes a wide excursion (> 10-15 mmHg) in the intracardiac pressure waveform. Intrathoracic pressure is significantly increased. As a result, the end-expiratory intracardiac pressure measurements will be artificially high. Measures to decrease the respiratory variation are helpful.

- Mechanical ventilators raise the intrathoracic pressure especially when PEEP is used. PEEP levels > 10 cm H_2O artificially raise bedside intracardiac pressure measurements. High levels of PEEP may also block retrograde transmission of the left atrial pressure events to the pulmonary capillary bed.

Chapter 2 References

1. Shabetai R. *The pericardium.* New York: Grune & Stratton. 1981;pp 81-107.

2. Leatherman JW, Marini J. Pulmonary artery catheter: pressure monitoring. In: Sprung CL, ed. *The Pulmonary Artery Catheter.* Closter, NJ: Critical Care Research Associates, Inc., 1993;pp 119-156.

3. Tuman KJ, Caroll GC, Ivankovich AD. Pitfalls in interpretation of pulmonary artery catheter data. *Journal of Cardiothorac Anesthesia* 1989;3:625-641.

4. West JB, Dollery CT, Naimark A. Distribution of pulmonary blood flow in isolated lung: Relation to vascular and alveolar pressures. *J Appl Physiol* 1964;19:713-724.

5. Shasby DM, Dauber IM, Pfister S, Anderson JT, Carson SB, Manart F, Hyers TM. Swan-Ganz catheter location and left atrial pressure determines the accuracy of the wedge pressure when positive end-expiratory pressure is used. *Chest* 1981;80:666-670.

6. Quinn R, Marini JJ. Pulmonary artery occlusion pressure; clinical physiology, measurement, and interpretation. *Am Rev Respir Dis* 1983;128:319-326.

7. Marini J, O'Quinn R, Culver BW, Butler J. Estimation of transmural cardiac pressures during ventilation with PEEP. *J Appl Physiol* 1982;53:384-391.

8. Buda AJ, Pinsky MR, Ingels NB, Daughters GT, Stinson EB, Alderman EL. Effect of intrathoracic pressure on left ventricular performance. *N Engl J Med* 1979;301:453-459.

9. Cohn JN, Hamosh P. Experimental observations in pulsus paradoxus and hepatojugular reflux. In: Reddy PS, editor. *Pericardial Disease.* New York; Raven Press, 1982;249-258.

10. Altose MD. Pulmonary mechanics. In: Fishman AP, ed. *Pulmonary Diseases and Disorders* (2nd edition). New York: McGraw-Hill, 1988; p.171.

11. West JB. *Respiratory Physiology - The Essentials.* Baltimore: Williams & Wilkins. 1995;pp 89-116.

12. Rice DL, Awe RJ, Gaasch WH, Alexander JK, Jenkins DE. Wedge pressure measurements in obstructive pulmonary disease. *Chest* 1974;66:628-632.

13. Downs JB. A technique for direct measurement of intrapleural pressure. *Crit Care Med* 1976;4:207-210.

14. Gillespie DJ. Comparison of intraesophageal balloon pressure measurements with a nasogastric-esophageal balloon system in volunteers. *Amer Rev Resp Dis* 1982;126:583-592.

15. Schuster DP, Seeman MD. Temporary muscle paralysis for accurate measurement of pulmonary artery occlusion pressure. *Chest* 1983;84:593-597.

16. Pick RA, Handler JB, Friedman AS. The cardiovascular effects of positive end-expiratory pressure. *Chest* 1982;82:345-350.

17. Pepe PE, Marini JJ. Occult positive end-expiratory pressure in mechanically ventilated patients with airflow obstruction. *Am Rev Respir Dis* 1982;126:166-170.

18. Jardin F, Genevray B, Brun-Ney D, Bourdarias JP. Influence of lung and chest wall compliances on transmission of airway pressure to the pleural space in critically ill patients. *Chest* 1985;86:653-658.

19. Craven KD, Wood LDH. Extrapericardial and esophageal pressures with positive end-expiratory pressure in dogs. *J Appl Physiol* 1981;51:798-805.

20. De Campo T, Civetta JM. The effect of short-term discontinuation of high-level PEEP in patients with acute respiratory failure. *Crit Care Med* 1979;7:47-49.

CARDIAC OUTPUT

The cardiac output can be measured in the Cardiac Care Unit using either the Thermodilution Method or the Fick Method. Both methods require a pulmonary artery catheter. Thermodilution is currently the most widely used method for the measurement of the cardiac output.

The Cardiac Output

The cardiac output is usually expressed in liters/minute. The cardiac index is obtained by dividing the cardiac output by the patient's body surface area:

$$\text{Cardiac Index} = \frac{\text{Cardiac Output}}{\text{Body Surface Area}}$$

The normal cardiac index is 2.6 - 4.2 L/min/m^2.

The cardiac output is the product of the heart rate and the stroke volume. It is important to measure the stroke volume because a change in the cardiac output may merely reflect a change in the patient's heart rate. The stroke volume index is calculated by dividing the stroke volume by the body surface area:

$$\text{Stroke Volume Index} = \frac{\text{Stroke Volume}}{\text{Body Surface Area}}$$

The normal stroke volume index is 30 - 65 mL/beat/m^2.

The right ventricular cardiac output (pulmonary blood flow) is measured by both the Fick and Thermodilution methods. With significant mitral or aortic valve regurgitation, the cardiac output of the left ventricle may greatly exceed that of the right ventricle. The volume of regurgitant blood cannot be measured with either the Fick or the thermodilution methods.

The systemic and pulmonary resistances can be calculated once the cardiac output and intracardiac pressure measurements have been recorded. The systemic vascular resistance (SVR) describes the relation between the mean arterial pressure and the cardiac output:

$$\text{SVR} = \frac{(\text{Mean Arterial Pressure - Right Atrial Pressure}) \times 80}{\text{Cardiac Output}}$$

The normal SVR = 700-1600 dynes-sec-cm^{-5}.

The total pulmonary resistance (TPR) describes the relation between the mean pulmonary artery pressure and the cardiac output:

$$\text{TPR} = \frac{\text{Mean Pulmonary Artery Pressure} \times 80}{\text{Cardiac Output}}$$

The normal TPR = 100-300 dynes-sec-cm^{-5}.

The pulmonary vascular resistance (PVR) measures the resistance to flow imposed by the lung vessels alone (without the influence of the left atrial pressure). This measurement is made by subtracting the wedge pressure (left atrial pressure) from the mean pulmonary artery pressure.

$$\text{PVR} = \frac{\left(\begin{array}{c} \text{Mean Pulmonary} \\ \text{Artery Pressure} \end{array} - \begin{array}{c} \text{Mean Wedge} \\ \text{Pressure} \end{array} \right) \times 80}{\text{Cardiac Output}}$$

The normal PVR = 20-130 dynes-sec-cm^{-5}.

It should be apparent that the accurate determination of these resistances requires precise measurement of the cardiac output, the systemic arterial pressure, the pulmonary artery pressure, the wedge pressure, and the right atrial pressure.

Thermodilution Method

The thermodilution method for the measurement of blood flow was introduced by Fegler in 1954.[1] Ganz *et. al.* refined the thermodilution method for use in the measurement of the cardiac output in patients and introduced it clinically in 1971.[2] The method is accurate, reproducible and can be performed repeatedly in critically ill patients.[3-5]

The thermodilution method is a form of the indicator-dilution technique.[6] The indicator in this case is cold solution injected into the right atrium through the proximal port of the pulmonary artery catheter. A thermistor near the catheter tip measures pulmonary artery temperature continuously. The thermistor is quite sensitive and can detect the changes in pulmonary artery temperature caused by breathing, (0.01 to 0.02°C).[7] After injection of the cold solution into the right atrium, the pulmonary artery temperature drops transiently. A thermodilution curve is generated by plotting the decline in the pulmonary artery temperature (°C) vs. time (seconds), *(Figure 3.1)*. The curve has a smooth steep upstroke and a slow decline to baseline. The area under the thermodilution curve is measured by the cardiac output computer. This is then incorporated into the Stewart-Hamilton equation to yield the cardiac output.[8] None of these calculations are apparent at the bedside since they are performed by the cardiac output computer. The operator only sees the cardiac output (liters/minute) flash on the screen. It is important for the operator to examine the thermodilution curve as a "check" on the computer generated number. The area under the thermodilution curve is inversely related to the cardiac output because the indicator (cold) is diluted by body temperature blood flow *(Figure 3.2)*.

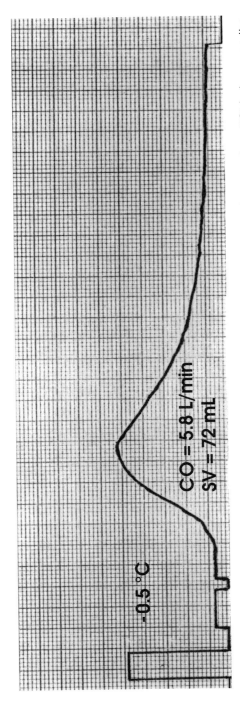

-0.5 °C

CO = 5.8 L/min
SV = 72 mL

Figure 3.1 Normal thermodilution cardiac output curve. Decline in pulmonary artery temperature (°C) is shown on the vertical axis versus time on the horizontal axis. After injection of 10 mL of iced solution, the pulmonary artery temperature drops suddenly, then gradually returns to the baseline. The area under this curve is inversely proportional to the cardiac output. CO = cardiac output, SV = stroke volume. Paper speed = 5 mm/sec. Calibration artifact = -0.5°C.

It is important to remember that the thermodilution method measures pulmonary blood flow. The pulmonary blood flow is nearly identical to the systemic blood flow unless a left to right shunt exists. For example, with a post-infarction ventricular septal defect, the pulmonary blood flow will exceed the systemic blood flow by an amount equal to the left to right shunt.

While the thermodilution method is quite accurate, the quality of the results are highly operator dependent.[8,9] All individuals performing the measurement must use a standardized procedure or the results will be inconsistent. The accuracy and reproducibility of the cardiac output measurement has been demonstrated with either ice temperature or room temperature injectates.[10] The following is a summary of the proper procedure for performing the thermodilution cardiac output:

1. Select the proper computation constant. This is specified by the catheter manufacturer and varies depending on the catheter type, the injectate temperature, and the injectate volume.

2. Inject the precise volume (usually 10 mL) over 2-4 seconds. Slight variations in the injectate volume will significantly alter results.

3. Note the heart rate and the rhythm during the injection and recording phase. The thermodilution method samples blood flow over a few seconds and extrapolates this to yield the blood flow per minute. A change in the heart rate or the rhythm during injection and recording will change the results.

4. When using iced solution, do not allow the injectate to warm before use. The solution should be withdrawn and injected within 15 seconds.

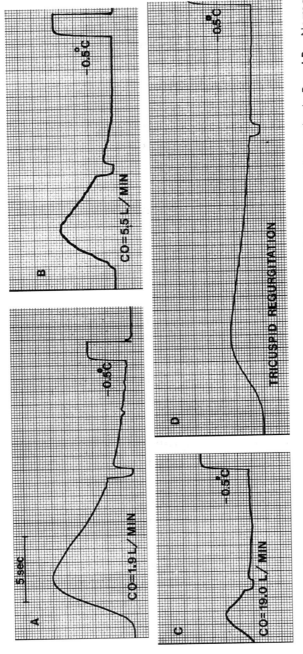

Figure 3.2 A spectrum of thermodilution cardiac output curves. **Panel A:** Low cardiac output. **Panel B:** Normal cardiac output. **Panel C:** High cardiac output. **Panel D:** Tricuspid regurgitation. The notches on the descending portion of the curves are artifacts generated by the cardiac output computer. Paper speed = 5 mm/sec.

5. The cardiac output measurements should vary by less than 10%. It is common for the first cardiac output measurement in a series to be higher than subsequent measurements. With the first injection, some of the indicator (cold) is lost as the catheter itself is cooled. The result is a smaller thermodilution curve. In this situation, the first measurement should be excluded. In general, the injections are performed in triplicate and averaged to yield the cardiac output measurement.

6. Finally, examine the thermodilution curve and place a representative example into the patient's chart.

Significant tricuspid regurgitation invalidates the thermodilution method because a portion of the indicator (cold) warms during its prolonged stay within the right atrium and right ventricle. Significant tricuspid regurgitation produces an easily identifiable thermodilution curve characterized by a very slow decay to baseline temperature *(Figures 3.2 and 3.3)*. The computer will measure the area under this curve and generate a "cardiac output" number. This measurement is unreliable and should be discarded.[11] Continuous measurement of the mixed venous oxygen saturation (pulmonary artery oxygen saturation) is especially useful in patients with severe tricuspid regurgitation[12] (described later in this chapter).

Some investigators recommend that serial cardiac output injections be performed at the same phase of respiration. Both the pulmonary artery temperature and the cardiac output vary with respiration.[9,13] Clearly, end-expiratory injections produce quite consistent results.[14] However, this process is somewhat tedious and may be impossible in patients with severe respiratory distress[9].

Fick Method

The Fick Method of cardiac output determination measures pulmonary blood flow using principles described by Adolph Fick

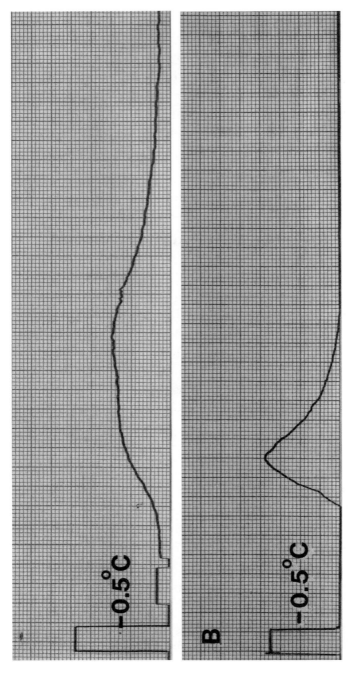

Figure 3.3 Thermodilution cardiac output curves from a patient with severe tricuspid regurgitation before (**top**) and after (**bottom**) tricuspid valve annuloplasty. At top, the upstroke of the curve is abnormally slow and the decay is prolonged due to the tricuspid regurgitation. The computer generated cardiac output would not be accurate. After repair of the tricuspid valve, the curve is normal. Paper speed = 5 mm/sec. Calibration artifact = -0.5 °C.

in 1870.[15] In the absence of a significant intracardiac shunt, the pulmonary blood flow and the systemic blood flow are equal. The Fick equation is:

$$\text{Cardiac Output (liters/minute)} = \frac{\text{Oxygen Consumption (mL of } O_2\text{/minute)}}{\text{Arteriovenous oxygen difference (mL of } O_2\text{/liter of blood)}}$$

An examination of this equation shows that the cardiac output varies inversely with the arteriovenous oxygen difference (AV O_2 difference) i.e. as the cardiac output decreases, the AV O_2 difference increases and vice versa. Precise measurement of the Fick cardiac output requires simultaneous determination of both oxygen consumption and AV O_2 difference. Cardiac output can be estimated by measuring only the AV O_2 difference and comparing it with a normal value. Serial measurement of the AV O_2 difference provides an estimate of the cardiac output over time.

AV O_2 Difference

An understanding of the AV O_2 difference is essential for proper use of the Fick cardiac output.[16] The AV O_2 difference is the amount of oxygen (mL) extracted by tissues from each liter of blood circulated. The AV O_2 difference requires measurement of the patient's hemoglobin, arterial oxygen percent saturation, and mixed venous oxygen percent saturation. The best source of a truly mixed venous blood sample is the pulmonary artery (a sample can easily be obtained by withdrawing blood from the distal lumen of the pulmonary artery catheter.) The AV O_2 difference calculation assumes that red cells with 100% oxygen saturation carry 1.36 mL of oxygen per gram of hemoglobin. The steps involved in the AV O_2 difference calculation are as follows:[17]

1. **Calculate the Arterial Oxygen Content.** Arterial oxygen content = Hemoglobin (gm/dL) x 10 (converts from deciliter to liter) x 1.36 (mL of O_2/gram of hemoglobin) x % arterial oxygen saturation. **Result** = mL of oxygen in each liter of arterial blood.

2. **Calculate the Mixed Venous Oxygen Content.** Mixed Venous (pulmonary artery) Oxygen Content = Hemoglobin (gm/dL) x 10 (converts from deciliter to liter) x 1.36 (mL of O_2/ gram of hemoglobin) x % pulmonary artery oxygen saturation. **Result** = mL of oxygen in each liter of mixed venous blood.

3. **Arteriovenous Oxygen Difference.** The arteriovenous oxygen difference = arterial oxygen content - mixed venous content. Please note that the first and second steps of the AV O_2 difference calculation involve redundancy (multiplication of hemoglobin x 10 x 1.36). Thus the AV O_2 difference calculation can be streamlined to:

AV O_2 difference = hemoglobin x 10 x 1.36 [% arterial oxygen saturation - % pulmonary artery oxygen saturation]

The normal arterial oxygen saturation is 93-98% and the normal pulmonary artery oxygen saturation is 75%. The normal resting AV O_2 difference is 30-50 mL of O_2/liter of blood (3.0-5.0 mL of O_2/100 mL of blood).[17]

Clinical Use of the AV O_2 Difference

The measurement of the AV O_2 difference provides the clinician with an *estimate* of the cardiac output. Serial measurement of the AV O_2 difference allows estimation of the cardiac output trend. Since the arterial oxygen saturation is usually constant, changes in the AV O_2 difference are usually the result of an increase or decrease in the mixed venous oxygen saturation. A decrease in the cardiac output is compensated by an increase in tissue oxygen extraction and a resultant decrease in the mixed venous saturation. For example, a patient faced with a 50% reduction in cardiac output maintains aerobic metabolism by doubling tissue oxygen extraction. In this example, the mixed venous oxygen saturation would drop from 75% to 50%. It is possible to easily measure mixed venous (pulmonary artery) oxygen saturation continuously using a pulmonary artery catheter equipped with fiberoptic bundles.[18] These catheters also allow conventional measurements of

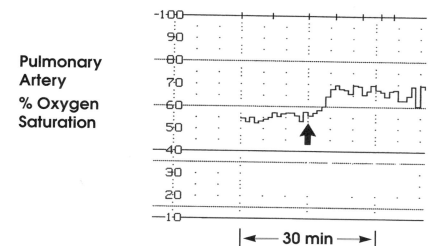

Pulmonary
Artery
% Oxygen
Saturation

|◄— 30 min —►|

Figure 3.4 Continuous measurement of mixed venous oxygen saturation through a pulmonary artery catheter in a patient with significant congestive failure. At baseline, the mixed venous saturation is reduced at 55%. After initiation of nitroprusside (bold arrow), the oxygen saturation increases reflecting an increase in cardiac output. min = minutes.

intracardiac pressure and the thermodilution cardiac output. Changes in mixed venous oxygen saturation reflect changes in the cardiac output provided that the patient's hemoglobin, arterial oxygen saturation, and oxygen consumption are all constant *(Figure 3.4)*. In a critically ill patient, these variables may be unstable and thus changes in pulmonary artery oxygen saturation must be interpreted carefully. Continuous measurement of the pulmonary artery oxygen saturation is helpful in selected critically ill patients especially when the thermodilution cardiac output measurement is invalid or yields unexpected results.

Oxygen Consumption

A precise measurement of the cardiac output using the Fick equation requires the additional measurement of the patient's oxygen consumption. In the past, this required collecting the patient's exhaled air over several minutes; not practical in the Intensive Care Unit. Fortunately, alternatives exist. First, bedside metabolic carts allow measurement of exhaled and inhaled air oxygen content using indirect calorimetry; this measurement requires scrupulous attention to detail.[19] Oxygen consumption per minute can be calculated from this data. Second, oxygen consumption can be assumed as basal (125 mL of O_2/min/m^2). Critically ill patients may actually consume more oxygen and this assumption may underestimate the cardiac output.

Sources of Error

The Fick Method makes many assumptions and requires several measurements. Common sources of error include:

- **Incorrect measurement of arterial or pulmonary artery blood % oxygen saturation.** Be sure that 2-3 mL of blood are withdrawn from any catheter and discarded before a sample is sent for measurement.

- **Peripheral shunting at the tissue level (septic shock).** Pulmonary artery blood may have a high oxygen saturation despite a low cardiac output.

- **Mitral or aortic regurgitation.** The Fick Method measures pulmonary blood flow. With significant mitral or aortic insufficiency, the total cardiac output of the left ventricle includes both forward blood flow (systemic blood flow) + regurgitant blood flow. In this situation, the pulmonary blood flow remains an accurate assessment of systemic blood flow but does not measure the volume of left ventricular regurgitation flow.

- **Intracardiac shunt.** With significant intracardiac shunting (atrial septal defect or ventricular septal defect), the pulmonary blood flow and systemic blood flow are no longer equal.

Key Points: Cardiac Output

- The cardiac output is the product of heart rate and stroke volume. A change in the cardiac output may reflect a change in the heart rate, stroke volume, or both.

- The cardiac output can be measured at the bedside using either the Thermodilution or the Fick methods. The thermodilution method is simpler and requires only measurement of the pulmonary artery blood temperature. The Fick method requires measurement of both the oxygen consumption and the arteriovenous oxygen difference.

- The cardiac output is inversely proportional to the area under the thermodilution curve. Significant tricuspid regurgitation invalidates the thermodilution method.

- The arteriovenous oxygen (AV O_2) difference measures tissue oxygen extraction. The AV O_2 difference is inversely proportional to the cardiac output.

- The mixed venous oxygen saturation (SV O_2) is an indicator of tissue oxygen extraction. The SV O_2 varies directly with the cardiac output. The SV O_2 can be measured continuously with a pulmonary artery catheter. The trend in the SV O_2 can be used to estimate the trend in the cardiac output.

Chapter 3 References

1. Fegler G. Measurement of cardiac output in anaesthetized animals by a thermodilution method. *QJ Exp Physiol* 1954;39:156-164.

2. Ganz W, Donoso R, Marcus HS, Forrester JS, Swan HJC. A new technique for measure-ment of cardiac output by thermodilution in man. *Am J Cardiol* 1971;27:392-396.

3. Levett JM, Replogle RL. Thermodilution cardiac output. A critical analysis and review of the literature. *J Surg Res* 1979;27:392-404.

4. Branthwaite MA, Bradley RD. Measurement of cardiac output by thermo-dilution in man. *J Appl Physiol* 1968;24:434-438.

5. Stetz CW, Miller RG, Kelly GE, Raffin TA. Reliability of the thermodilution method in determination of cardiac output in clinical practice. *Am Rev Respir Dis* 1982;126:1001-1004.

6. Weisel RD, Berger RL, Hechtman HB. Measurement of cardiac output by thermodilution. *N Engl J Med* 1975;292:682-684.

7. Ganz W, Swan HJC. Measurement of blood flow by thermodilution. *Am J Cardiol* 1972;29:241-245.

8. Kett DH, Schein RMH. Techniques for pulmonary artery catheter insertion. In: Sprung CL, editor. *The Pulmonary Artery Catheter*, 2nd ed. Closter: Critical Care Research Associates, Inc., 1993;69-72.

9. Tuman KJ, Carroll GC, Ivankovich AD. Pitfalls in interpretation of pulmonary artery catheter data. *J Cardiothoracic Anesth* 1989;3:625-541.

10. Elkayam U, Berkley R, Azen S, Weber L, Geva B, Henry WL. Cardiac output by thermodilution technique. Effect of injectate's volume and temperature on accuracy and reproducibility in the critically ill patient. *Chest* 1983;84:418-422.

11. Cigarroa RG, Lange RA, Williams RH, Bedoto JB, Hillis LD. Underestimation of cardiac output by thermodilution in patients with tricuspid regurgitation. *Am J Med* 1989;86:417-420.

12. Davies GG, Jebson PR, Glascow BM, Hess DR. Continuous Fick cardiac output compared to thermodilution cardiac output. *Crit Care Med* 1986;14:881-885.

13. Snyder JV, Powner DJ. Effects of mechanical ventilation on the measurement of cardiac output by thermodilution. *Crit Care Med* 1982;10:677-682.

14. Stevens JH, Raffin TA, Mihm FG, Rosenthal MH, Stetz CW. Thermodilution cardiac output measurement. Effects of the respiratory cycle on its reproducibility. *JAMA* 1985;253:2240-42.

15. Fick A. Uber die Messung des Blutquantums in den Herzventrikeln. Sitz der *Physik-Med Ges Wurtzberg* 1870;16.

16. Finch CA, Lenfant C. Oxygen transport in man. *N Engl J Med* 1972;286:407-415.

17. Grossman W, McLaurin LP. Clinical measurement of vascular resistance and assessment of vasodilator drugs. In: Grossman W, editor. *Cardiac Catheterization and Angiography*, 2nd ed. Philadelphia: Lea & Febiger, 1980;116-123.

18. Gore JM, Sloan K. Use of continuous monitoring of mixed venous saturation in the Coronary Care Unit. *Chest* 1984;86:757-761.

19. Makita K, Nunn JF. Evaluation of metabolic measuring instruments for use in critically ill patients. *Crit Care Med* 1990; 18:638-644.

ARRHYTHMIAS

The mechanical action of the heart is governed by the cardiac rhythm. An arrhythmia will therefore have an immediate impact on hemodynamic parameters. When analyzing this effect, it is important to consider the following:

- What is the arrhythmia rate?
- What is the effect of the arrhythmia on coordinated atrial-ventricular contraction (atrial-ventricular synchrony)?
- Has the arrhythmia compromised the efficiency of atrial or ventricular systole?

For example, atrial fibrillation excludes normal atrial contraction. Ventricular premature beats are less forceful because the normal pattern of ventricular depolarization is disrupted.[1] This chapter focuses on the changes in hemodynamic parameters that accompany a variety of common cardiac arrhythmias.

Sinus Tachycardia

With an increase in the heart rate, diastole progressively shortens. As a consequence, the A wave initiating a cardiac cycle begins to encroach on the V wave of the preceding cycle (*Figure 4.1, Panels A-C).* Eventually the two waves summate to generate a single

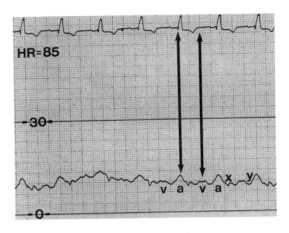

Figure 4.1 (Panels A-C) Right atrial pressure waveforms from a patient at 3 different heart rates. The PR interval is normal.

Panel A: Sinus rhythm at 85 beats/min. Normal A(**a**) and V (**v**) waves with X (**x**) and Y descents (**y**) present.

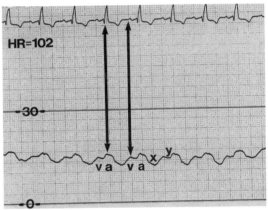

Panel B: Sinus rhythm at 102 beats/min. The A wave (**a**) begins to blend with the V wave (**v**) of the preceding cardiac cycle. As a result, the Y descent (**y**) is attenuated. This should not be confused with the absent Y descent of pericardial tamponade.

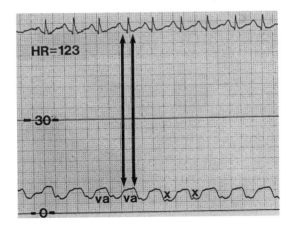

Panel C: Sinus rhythm at 123 beats/min. The A wave (**a**) has now fused with the V wave (**v**) of the preceding cardiac cycle. The Y descent is absent.

HR = heart rate;
Scale = 0-30 mmHg;
Paper speed = 25 mm/sec.

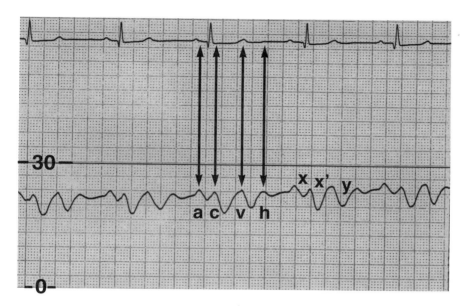

Figure 4.2 Right atrial pressure waveform from a patient with sinus bradycardia at 49 beats/min. An H wave (**h**) is present due to the long diastole. The A-C interval is slightly prolonged due to first degree AV block. The right atrial pressure is elevated (21 mmHg) in this patient with inferior/right ventricular infarction. The H wave is accentuated when the right atrial pressure is elevated. HR = heart rate; Scale = 0-30 mmHg; Paper speed = 25 mm/sec.

wave and the Y descent is obliterated *(Figure 4.1)*. It is important to remember the influence of heart rate on the Y descent because pericardial tamponade also causes disappearance of the Y descent *(Chapter 11)*. First degree AV block can cause the A and V waves to summate in the same way as does sinus tachycardia. Therefore, both the heart rate and the PR interval must be considered when evaluating the atrial pressure waveforms.

Sinus Bradycardia

As diastole lengthens during sinus bradycardia, the time interval lengthens between the V wave of one cardiac cycle and the A wave of the next cycle. The Y descent is easily seen *(Figure 4.2)*. Often an additional positive wave (the H wave) is present after the Y descent when the heart rate is less than 60 beats/min *(Figure 4.2)*. This

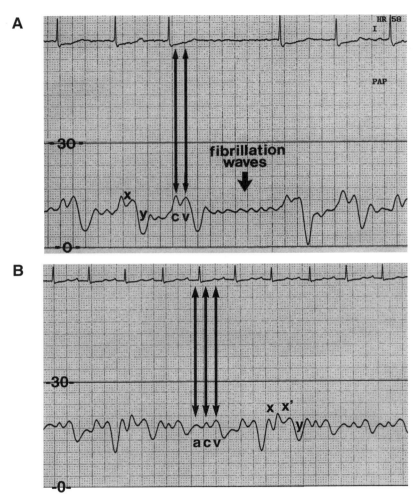

Figure 4.3 (Panels A & B) Right atrial pressure waveforms from a patient during atrial fibrillation and after spontaneous conversion to sinus rhythm.
Panel A: During atrial fibrillation, the C (**c**) and V waves (**v**) are dominant due to loss of the A wave. Fibrillation waves can be seen during the diastole accompanying a long R-R interval. The Y descent (**y**) is steeper than the X descent (**x**) as is typical of atrial fibrillation. The right atrial pressure is elevated (10 mmHg) in this patient with inferior/right ventricular infarction.
Panel B: Right atrial pressure waveform from the same patient after conversion to sinus rhythm. The A wave (**a**) has returned.
Scale = 0-30 mmHg; Paper speed = 25 mm/sec.

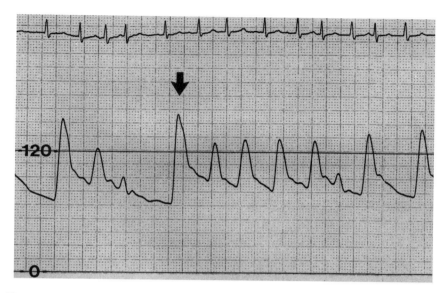

Figure 4.4 Systemic arterial pressure waveform during atrial fibrillation. The arterial pulse pressure varies directly with the R-R interval. Following long R-R intervals, the ventricular stroke volume and therefore the arterial pulse pressure increase (**arrow**). Scale = 0-120 mmHg; Paper speed = 25 mm/sec.

wave is most prominent in the right atrial pressure waveform especially when the right atrial pressure is elevated.[2] The origin of the H wave is unclear and is not associated with any mechanical cardiac event.[3]

Atrial Fibrillation

The hallmarks of atrial fibrillation are disappearance of atrial systole and variation in the length of diastole. The A wave disappears from the atrial pressure waveform and is sometimes replaced by atrial fibrillation waves (*Figure 4.3*). The fibrillation waves are most evident during a long R-R interval. These waves are sometimes visible in the jugular veins and can produce enough mechanical activity to move the mitral and tricuspid valves.[4] The fibrillation waves are associated with coarse atrial fibrillation on the electrocardiogram. The C and V waves are

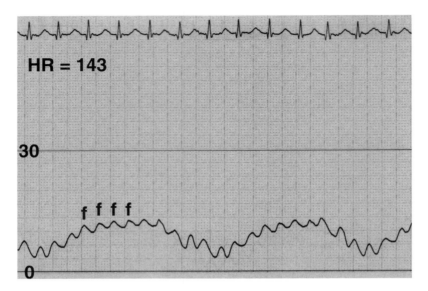

Figure 4.5 Right atrial pressure waveform from a patient with atrial flutter demonstrates typical mechanical flutter waves (**f**). The atrial rate is somewhat less than 300 beats/min because of treatment with a type IA antiarrhythmic drug. Scale = 0-30 mmHg; Paper speed = 25 mm/sec.

dominant features of the atrial pressure waveform. The C and V waves are separated by the X descent. The X descent is usually shallower than the Y descent[5,6] *(Figure 4.3)*. Many patients with atrial fibrillation have coexisting myocardial or pericardial disease and the atrial pressure waveform may also be influenced by these pathological conditions. During atrial fibrillation, the ventricular stroke volume varies directly with the electrocardiographic R-R interval. As a result, the pulse pressure in the aorta and the pulmonary artery will be greatest following a long R-R interval *(Figure 4.4)*.

Atrial Flutter

As with atrial fibrillation, the A wave of the atrial pressure waveform is absent. During atrial flutter, the atria continue to contract at a rate of approximately 300 beats/min. This mechanical atrial activity generates flutter waves in the atrial pressure waveform[4,7] *(Figure 4.5)*. This regular mechanical activity

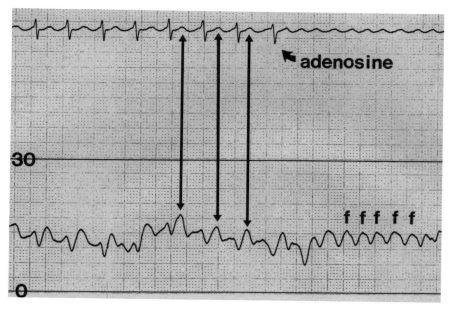

Figure 4.6 Right atrial pressure waveform from a patient with atrial flutter and 2:1 AV conduction. At left, alternate flutter waves are exaggerated (**arrows**) because they occur during ventricular systole. At right, an adenosine bolus transiently induces complete heart block. All flutter waves (**f**) are now monomorphic because of absent ventricular systole. Scale = 0-30 mmHg; Paper speed = 25 mm/sec.

may partly explain why the systemic embolism rate during atrial flutter is lower than during atrial fibrillation. In the presence of 2:1 AV block, every other flutter wave often occurs coincident with ventricular systole. The flutter waves occurring during ventricular systole may be slightly enhanced because the right atrium is contracting against a closed tricuspid valve *(Figure 4.6)*.

Premature Ventricular Contractions

A premature ventricular contraction sets the stage for a mechanical cannon wave (cannon A wave). Cannon waves are the result of an atrial systole occurring when ventricular systole has already closed the mitral and tricuspid valves *(Figure 4.7)*. That is, atrial and ventricular systole are either simultaneous or reversed from their normal timing sequence. The cannon wave

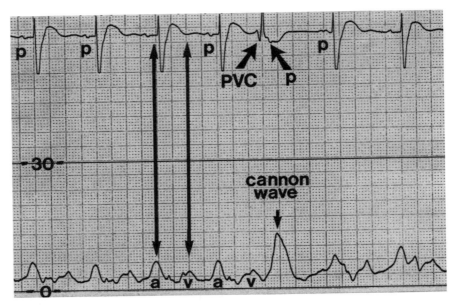

Figure 4.7 Right atrial pressure waveform during sinus rhythm with a single premature ventricular contraction (**PVC**). The sinus P wave (**p**) is clearly visible in the ST segment of the PVC. The normal sequence of atrial-ventricular systole is reversed and a cannon wave results.
Scale = 0-30 mmHg; Paper speed = 25 mm/sec.

causes a transient reversal in the normal systemic and pulmonary venous return.[8] The ventricles are not properly filled at the onset of systole. Isolated premature ventricular contractions rarely disturb overall cardiac performance. The astute examiner will learn to recognize the characteristic appearance of the cannon wave. A cannon wave in the atrial pressure waveform is a helpful marker that the normal sequence of atrial and ventricular systole has been disturbed. Cannon waves can be seen with a variety of arrhythmias described later in this chapter.

AV Junctional (Nodal) Rhythm

During a nodal rhythm, atrial systole can either precede or follow ventricular systole. AV dissociation may also occur. When the sequence of atrial and ventricular systole is reversed, cannon waves will be present on the atrial pressure waveform (*Figure 4.8*).

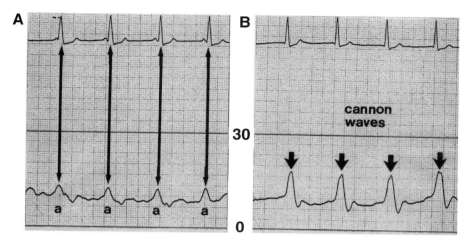

Figure 4.8 (Panels A & B) Right atrial pressure waveforms from a patient during nodal rhythm.
Panel A: The sinus rate and the nodal rate are nearly the same (Isorhythmic dissociation). The P wave precedes the QRS complex and the normal sequence of atrial-ventricular systole is maintained. A normal right atrial A wave (**a**) is present.
Panel B: The P wave now occurs within the QRS complex. Atrial and ventricular systole are nearly simultaneous which generates cannon waves (**arrows**) in the right atrial pressure tracing.
Scale = 0-30 mmHg; Paper speed = 25 mm/sec.

AV Nodal Reentrant Tachycardia

Reentry within the AV node is one of the most common causes of paroxysmal supraventricular tachycardia.[9] Each time the electrical impulse travels the reentrant loop, there is retrograde activation of the atria and antegrade activation of the ventricles. In the majority of patients with this arrhythmia, the retrograde P wave occurs either within or after the QRS complex.[10] When ventricular systole is coincident with atrial systole, the A and V waves fuse and cannon waves occur[11] *(Figure 4.9)*. The cannon waves are regular because there is 1:1 AV association *(Figure 4.9)*. Patients may sense these right atrial cannon waves as pounding in the neck.[12] The cannon waves also abruptly elevate the right atrial mean pressure[11] *(Figures 4.9 & 4.10)*. This abrupt increase in right atrial pressure can trigger the release of atrial natriuretic

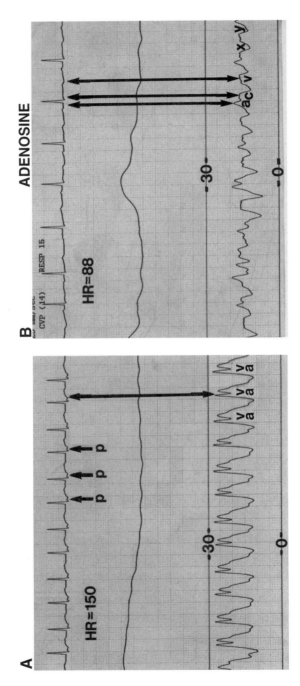

Figure 4.9 (Panels A & B) Right atrial pressure waveforms during reentrant supraventricular tachycardia and after conversion to sinus rhythm.

Panel A: Reentrant supraventricular tachycardia at a rate of 150 beats/min. Retrograde P waves (**p**) are visible at the end of the QRS complex. The normal sequence of atrial-ventricular systole is reversed which generates regular cannon waves (**v/a**) in the right atrial pressure tracing. The mean right atrial pressure is elevated at 19 mmHg.

Panel B: Intravenous adenosine restores sinus rhythm. Normal A (**a**), C (**c**), and V waves (**v**) are now present. The mean right atrial pressure has abruptly dropped to 13 mmHg.

HR = heart rate; Scale = 0-30 mmHg; Paper speed = 25 mm/sec.

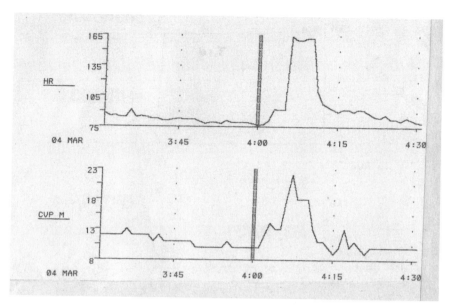

Figure 4.10 Graphic presentation of the change in heart rate (**HR**) and mean central venous pressure (**CVP M**) that occur with the onset of reentrant supraventricular tachycardia. At baseline, the heart rate is 76 beats/min and the mean central venous pressure is 10 mmHg. During tachycardia, the heart rate is 165 beats/min and the mean central venous pressure is 23 mmHg.

factor and may be responsible for polyuria in some of these patients.[13] The forward stroke volume, aortic systolic blood pressure, and aortic pulse pressure are often reduced during this tachycardia because of the shortened diastole coupled with the loss of the normal atrial contribution to ventricular filling[11] *(Figure 4.11)*. In some patients, the cannon waves may trigger a vasodepressor reflex further aggravating the fall in blood pressure.[14] Termination of the tachycardia usually restores hemodynamic parameters to normal immediately *(Figure 4.11)*.

Automatic Atrial Tachycardia

This arrhythmia is due to enhanced atrial automaticity. The atrial rate is usually less than 200 beats/min and generates rapid regular A waves in the atrial pressure waveform. It is common to observe

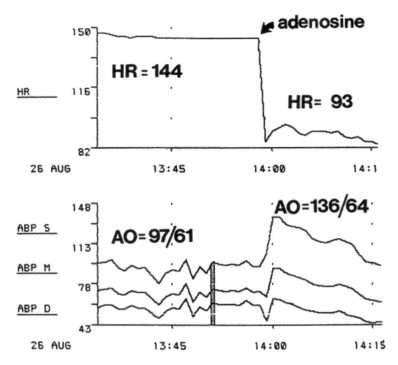

Figure 4.11 Graphic representation of the change in heart rate (**HR**) and arterial blood pressure (**ABP**) systolic (**S**), mean (**M**), diastolic (**D**) after conversion of reentrant supraventricular tachycardia to sinus rhythm. The systolic blood pressure rises 39 mmHg and the pulse pressure rises 36 mmHg due to an increase in the stroke volume with restoration of sinus rhythm.

2:1 AV nodal block.[15] In this circumstance, the blocked P wave usually occurs within the QRS-T interval. The A wave of the blocked P wave sums with the V wave of the QRS complex creating a single larger wave *(Figure 4.12)*. This "summation" wave does not have the appearance of a typical cannon wave perhaps because it occurs at the very end of ventricular systole near the time when tricuspid and mitral valve opening occur.

Ventricular Tachycardia

Ventricular tachycardia arises within the ventricles. Atrial activation occurs either by coexisting sinus rhythm (AV dissociation) or by retrograde VA conduction to the atria (VA

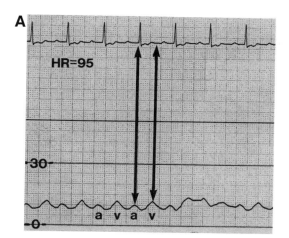

Figure 4.12 Panel A: Right atrial pressure waveform and lead II electrocardiogram resemble sinus rhythm. However, the right atrial V wave (**v**) is noticeably higher than the A wave (**a**)

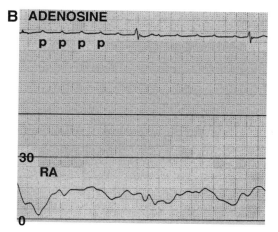

Panel B: Administration of adenosine reveals that the rhythm is actually an automatic atrial tachycardia at a rate of about 200 beats/min. The right atrial pressure waveform in Panel A is actually distorted. The V waves seen in Panel A are being augmented by the A waves of the atrial tachycardia.
RA = right atrium;
Scale = 0-30 mmHg;
Paper speed = 25 mm/sec.

association).[16] The type of atrial electrical activation has an important influence on the hemodynamic consequences of ventricular tachycardia.

With AV dissociation, the relation between atrial and ventricular systole is random. On some cycles, ventricular systole precedes atrial systole and cannon waves occur in the atrial pressure waveform. These beats generate a reduced stroke volume and therefore a reduced aortic pulse pressure because of absent atrial filling of the ventricles *(Figures 4.13 & 4.14)*. On other cycles, atrial systole precedes ventricular systole (mimicking normal physiology) and cannon waves are absent on the atrial

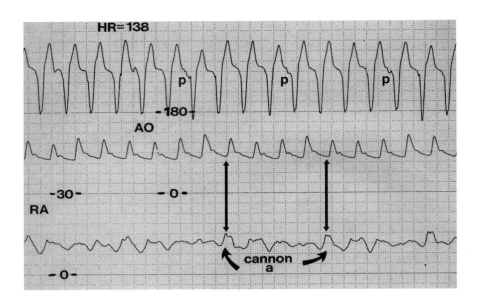

Figure 4.13 Right atrial (**RA**) and aortic (**AO**) pressure waveforms from a patient with ventricular tachycardia and AV dissociation. Irregular cannon waves due to a reversed sequence of atrial-ventricular contraction are present in the right atrial tracing. Because of poor ventricular filling, these beats produce a lower stroke volume and therefore a lower pulse pressure (**arrows**). Occasionally, the P waves (**p**) precede the QRS complex and the normal sequence of atrial-ventricular systole occurs. Cannon waves are absent on these beats and the aortic pulse pressure is wider because of improved stroke volume. HR = heart rate; Scale = 0-180 mmHg (AO) and 0-30 mmHg (RA); Paper speed = 25 mm/sec.

pressure waveform. These beats generate an improved stroke volume and therefore a higher aortic pulse pressure because atrial systole augments ventricular filling *(Figures 4.13 & 4.14)*. Physical examination of these patients reveals irregular cannon waves in the jugular venous pulse as well as a variable carotid artery pulse volume despite a regular cardiac rhythm.

With 1:1 VA conduction during ventricular tachycardia, the normal sequence of atrial and ventricular contraction is reversed on every cycle. Regular cannon waves appear in the atrial pressure waveform and the aortic pulse pressure remains constant

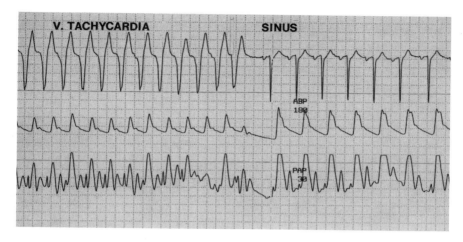

Figure 4.14 Arterial (**ABP**) and pulmonary artery (**PAP**) pressure waveforms from a patient with ventricular tachycardia and AV dissociation. Spontaneous conversion to sinus rhythm occurred during the recording. During ventricular tachycardia the arterial pulse pressure is reduced reflecting a low stroke volume. In addition, there is variation in the arterial pulse pressure due to AV dissociation. With conversion to sinus rhythm, the arterial pulse pressure immediately increases due to an improved stroke volume. V. tachycardia = ventricular tachycardia; Scale = 0-180 mmHg (ABP) and 0-30 mmHg (PAP); Paper speed = 25 mm/sec.

from beat to beat *(Figure 4.15)*. In these patients regular cannon waves are present in the jugular venous pulse and the carotid artery pulse volume is constant.

 Key Points: Arrhythmias

- Sinus tachycardia shortens diastole resulting in the summation of the A wave of one beat with the V wave of the previous beat. Prolongation of the PR interval has a similar effect.

- Atrial fibrillation results in the loss of the A wave with the appearance of fibrillatory waves. With atrial flutter, the A wave is replaced by flutter waves.

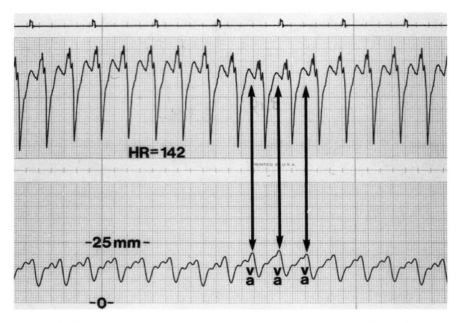

Figure 4.15 Right atrial pressure waveform from a patient with ventricular tachycardia and 1:1 VA conduction. Regular cannon waves (**v/a**) are present on the right atrial pressure tracing.
HR = heart rate; Scale = 0-25 mmHg; Paper speed = 25 mm/sec.

- The cannon A wave signals a reversal in the normal cardiac contraction sequence; ventricular systole precedes atrial systole. Cannon waves are observed in a variety of arrhythmias.

- With reentrant supraventricular tachycardias ventricular systole often precedes atrial systole. Consequently, regular cannon waves are observed in the atrial pressure waveforms. These cannon waves raise the mean atrial pressures.

- With ventricular tachycardia, the sequence of atrial and ventricular contraction is either random (AV dissociation) or reversed (VA conduction). With AV dissociation, irregular cannon waves are present. With VA conduction, regular cannon waves are present.

- Careful examination of the aortic pulse pressure can be used to deduce the effect of an arrhythmia on left ventricular stroke volume.

Chapter 4 References

1. Wiggers CJ. *The Pressure Pulses in the Cardiovascular System*. London: Longmans, Green and Co., 1928: 170.

2. Mackay I. The true venous pulse wave, central and peripheral. *Am Heart J* 1967;74:48-57.

3. Mackay I, Walker RL. An experimental examination of factors responsible for the 'h' (d") wave of the jugular phlebogram in human beings. *Am Heart J* 1966; 71:228-239.

4. Fujii J, Foster JR, Mills PG, Moos S, Craige E. Dual echocardiographic determination of atrial contraction sequence in atrial flutter and other related atrial arrhythmias. *Circulation* 1978; 58:314-321.

5. Wood P. *Disease of the Heart and Circulation*, 2nd ed. Philadelphia: JB Lippincott Co., 1962: 583.

6. Cairns KB, Kloster FE, Bristow JD, Lees MH, Griswold HE. Problems in the hemodynamic diagnosis of tricuspid insufficiency. *Am Heart J* 1968; 75:173-179.

7. Hatle L, Angelsen B. *Doppler Ultrasound in Cardiology*, 2nd ed. Philadelphia: Lea & Febiger, 1985: 275.

8. Naito M, Dreifus LS, David D, Michelson EL, Mardelli TJ, Kmetzo JJ. Reevaluation of the role of atrial systole to cardiac hemodynamics: evidence for pulmonary venous regurgitation during abnormal atrioventricular sequencing. *Am Heart J* 1983; 105:295-302.

9. Josephson ME, Kastor JA. Supraventricular tachycardia: mechanisms and management. *Ann Intern Med* 1977; 87:346-358.

10. Zipes DP. Specific arrhythmias: diagnosis and treatment. In: Braunwald E, editor. *Heart Disease: A Textbook of Cardiovascular Medicine*, 3rd ed. Philadelphia: WB Saunders, 1988: 681.

11. Goldreyer BN, Kastor JA, Kershbaum KL. The hemodynamic effects of induced supra-ventricular tachycardia in man. *Circulation* 1976; 54:783-789.

12. Gürsoy S, Steurer G, Brugada J, Andries E, Brugada P. Brief Report: The hemodynamic mechanism of pounding in the neck in atrioventricular nodal reentrant tachycardia. *N Engl J Med* 1992; 327:772-774.

13. Yamaji T, Ismibasi M, Nakaoka H, Imataka K, Amano M, Fujii J. Possible role for atrial natriuretic peptide in polyuria associated with paroxysmal atrial arrhythmias. *Lancet* 1985; 1:1211..

14. Erlebacher JA, Danner RL, Stelzer PE. Hypotension with ventricular pacing: an atrial vasodepressor reflex in human beings. *J Am Coll Cardiol* 1984; 4:550-555.

15. Zipes DP. Specific arrhythmias: diagnosis and treatment. In: Braunwald E, editor. *Heart Disease: A Textbook of Cardiovascular Medicine*, 3rd ed. Philadelphia: WB Saunders, 1988: 674-675.

16. Zipes DP. Specific arrhythmias: diagnosis and treatment. In: Braunwald E, editor. *Heart Disease: A Textbook of Cardiovascular Medicine*, 3rd ed. Philadelphia: WB Saunders, 1988: 694.

5

ACUTE MITRAL REGURGITATION
AND THE V WAVE

A cute mitral valve regurgitation is a catastrophic event occurring as a result of ruptured chordae tendinae, ruptured papillary muscle, or bacterial destruction of the mitral valve. The clinical diagnosis of acute mitral regurgitation is challenging; the murmur is atypical and often difficult to hear because of tachycardia, hypotension, and respiratory distress.[1] The severity and time course of the valvular insufficiency both have a major impact on the hemodynamic consequences of acute mitral regurgitation.[2] Chronic mitral regurgitation may be severe with little or no change in the bedside hemodynamic measurements and will not be discussed.[3]

Wedge Pressure & Pulmonary Artery Pressure

With acute mitral valve regurgitation, the left ventricle ejects blood into the left atrium during systole. The left atrium is subjected to an acute volume overload because the high pressure regurgitant volume is added to the normal pulmonary venous return. When the left ventricle is ejecting blood into a normal-sized and relatively unyielding left atrium, the wedge pressure (left atrial pressure) rises dramatically during ventricular systole. Mitral regurgitation begins with the onset of left ventricular systole (marked by the C wave in the wedge pressure waveform) and continues until the end of systole (marked by the peak of the V wave in the wedge pressure waveform). The hallmark of acute mitral regurgitation is a giant "C-V" wave in the wedge pressure tracing. The X' descent which normally separates the C wave from the V wave disappears or is attenuated. This "C-V" wave is therefore commonly referred to as simply the V wave *(Figure 5.1)*. The large V wave causes a striking increase in the mean wedge pressure *(Figure 5.1)*. The mean wedge pressure frequently exceeds 25-30 mmHg resulting in acute pulmonary edema.

The giant V wave of acute mitral regurgitation may be transmitted retrogradely into the pulmonary artery.[4,5] This yields a bifid pulmonary artery systolic waveform composed of the pulmonary artery systolic wave followed shortly by the V wave *(Figure 5.1)*. As the catheter moves from the pulmonary artery position into the wedge position, the pulmonary artery systolic wave disappears and only the V wave remains *(Figure 5.1)*. The wedge pressure V wave may be so striking as to resemble the pulmonary artery systolic pressure waveform and the operator may not realize that the catheter has moved from the pulmonary artery into the wedge position *(Figure 5.1)*. This problem can be avoided by carefully examining the pulmonary artery pressure waveform and its relation to the electrocardiogram. The timing of the peak pulmonary artery systolic wave and the peak V wave are significantly different. The pulmonary artery systolic wave occurs at the peak of the electrocardiographic T wave; the V wave occurs after the T wave *(Figure 5.1)*. The transient reversal of pulmonary blood flow that accompanies the giant V wave can result in highly oxygenated blood entering the main pulmonary artery resulting in the mistaken diagnosis of a left-to-right shunt.[6]

The wedge pressure A wave is not significantly changed by acute mitral regurgitation unless an arrhythmia such as atrial fibrillation complicates the situation *(Chapter 4)*.

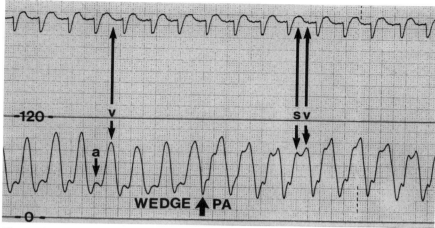

Figure 5.1 Wedge pressure and pulmonary artery pressure waveforms from a patient with acute severe mitral regurgitation. The wedge pressure waveform is shown first and is dominated by a large V wave (**v**). The mean wedge pressure is 54 mmHg and the V wave peak is 95 mmHg. The giant V wave causes the wedge pressure waveform to resemble that of an artery. The balloon is deflated (**large arrow**) to reveal the pulmonary artery (**PA**) pressure waveform. Severe pulmonary hypertension (91/34 mmHg) is present. The pulmonary artery systolic waveform is bifid and composed of the pulmonary artery systolic wave (**s**) followed shortly by the retrogradely transmitted giant V wave. The V wave in this patient is higher than the pulmonary artery systolic wave. This retrograde V wave should not be confused with the dicrotic wave of pulmonic valve closure. The timing of the wedge pressure V wave is identical to that of the pulmonary artery V wave. Note also that the pulmonary artery diastolic pressure (34 mmHg) under-estimates the mean wedge pressure (54 mmHg). The best method to estimate the left ventricular filling pressure in this patient would be to measure the wedge pressure at the end of the A wave (40mmHg).
Scale = 0-120 mmHg; Paper speed = 25 mm/sec.

Right Atrial Pressure

As would be expected, the right atrial pressure is of little clinical value in the setting of acute mitral insufficiency. The right atrial pressure A wave may be augmented because of pulmonary hypertension. Tricuspid regurgitation *(Chapter 6)* may occur if right ventricular failure occurs. When acute mitral regurgitation complicates inferior-right ventricular infarction, the right atrial pressure waveform may show features of right ventricular infarction *(Chapter 8)*.

Cardiac Output & Aortic Pressure

The cardiac output is decreased and shock is frequently present.[2] The left ventricular forward stroke volume (i.e., blood ejected across the aortic valve) is decreased.[2] Sinus tachycardia compensates to some degree for the decreased forward stroke volume. The total left ventricular stroke volume (blood ejected into the left atrium plus blood ejected across the aortic valve) may be normal. The aortic systolic pressure is usually low. The aortic pulse pressure is usually narrow reflecting a decreased left ventricular forward stroke volume. The thermodilution cardiac output method measures the pulmonary blood flow which is the same as the forward flow across the aortic valve. The thermodilution method therefore ignores the volume of blood ejected into the left atrium. This cannot be measured at the bedside with hemodynamic techniques.

General Comments on the V Wave

Several comments regarding the wedge pressure V wave are relevant to this chapter. The V wave is a normal finding on the wedge pressure tracing and is often higher than the A wave. Therefore, the definition of a "large" V wave is subjective. Furthermore, a large V wave commonly occurs in conditions other than acute mitral regurgitation. For example, prominent V waves are often observed with left ventricular failure from any cause (i.e., dilated cardiomyopathy, ischemic cardiomyopathy).[7,8] These prominent V waves may occur in the absence of significant mitral regurgitation and are usually a marker for a distended and noncompliant left atrium[7,8] (*Figure 5.2*). An acute ventricular septal defect (complicating myocardial infarction) can cause a large V wave because of the increased pulmonary blood flow and increased pulmonary venous return to the left atrium.[9] It should be apparent that a large V wave in the wedge pressure waveform must be interpreted carefully and in the context of the patient's clinical status.

Mitral regurgitation is often a dynamic event and the magnitude of the V wave may therefore vary considerably over time.[10] This is especially true during episodes of acute myocardial ischemia[11-13]

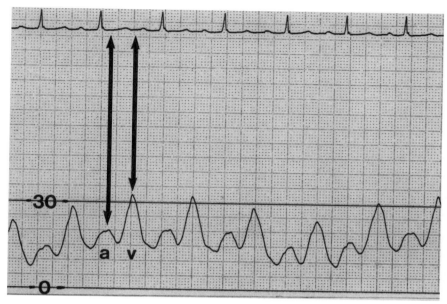

Figure 5.2 Wedge pressure waveform from a patient with dilated cardiomyopathy. The mean wedge pressure is elevated at 20 mmHg. A large V wave (**v**) is present and measures 32 mmHg. Doppler echocardiography revealed only mild mitral regurgitation. Scale = 0-30 mmHg;Paper speed = 25 mm/sec.

(Chapter 9). The degree of mitral regurgitation is sensitive to left ventricular afterload. Afterload reduction with nitroglycerin or nitroprusside can significantly reduce the amount of mitral regurgitation and the size of the wedge pressure V wave[14] *(Figure 5.3, Panels A & B).*

A large V wave disrupts the normal close correlation between the pulmonary artery diastolic pressure and the mean wedge pressure. The pulmonary artery diastolic pressure is a measurement made at a single point in time (end diastole), while the wedge pressure is a mean pressure recorded over the entire cardiac cycle. The peaks and valleys of a normal wedge pressure waveform are minor, therefore the pulmonary artery diastolic pressure usually correlates closely with the mean wedge pressure *(Chapter 1).* A large V wave distorts the wedge pressure waveform

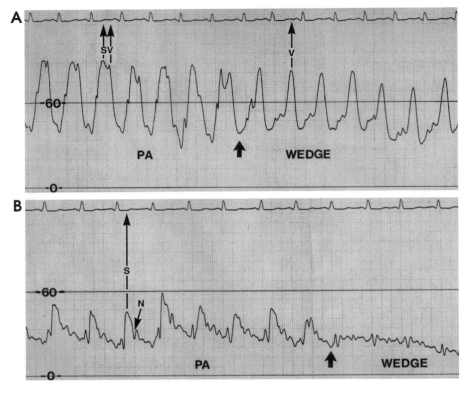

Figure 5.3 (Panels A & B) Pulmonary artery and wedge pressure waveforms from a patient with acute severe mitral regurgitation before and after treatment with intravenous nitroglycerin.

Panel A: Before nitroglycerin, severe pulmonary hypertension (95/41 mmHg) is present. The pulmonary artery (**PA**) systolic waveform is bifid and composed of the pulmonary artery systolic wave (**S**) and the retrograde V wave (**V**). The retrograde V wave is slightly less than the pulmonary artery systolic wave. The balloon is inflated (**large arrow**) to reveal the wedge pressure waveform. The wedge pressure waveform is dominated by the large V wave. The timing of the wedge pressure V wave is identical to that of the pulmonary artery V wave. The mean wedge pressure is 57 mmHg while the V wave peak is 80 mmHg. The pulmonary artery diastolic pressure (41 mmHg) underestimates the mean wedge pressure (57 mmHg).

Panel B: Minutes after treatment with intravenous nitroglycerin, the pulmonary artery pressure has dropped to 47/23 mmHg and the mean wedge pressure has dropped to 24 mmHg. The large V wave has disappeared from both the pulmonary artery and the wedge pressure waveforms. A normal dicrotic notch (**N**) and dicrotic wave are visible in the pulmonary artery pressure waveform. The pulmonary artery diastolic pressure (23 mmHg) now correlates closely with the mean wedge pressure (24 mmHg). The heart rate has decreased from 96 to 84 beats/min.

Scale = 0-60 mmHg; Paper speed = 25 mm/sec.

so that the pulmonary artery diastolic pressure now underestimates the mean wedge pressure *(Figures 5.1 & 5.3, Panel A)*. Consequently, the pulmonary artery diastolic pressure cannot be used as an estimate of the mean wedge pressure in the presence of a large V wave. As a corollary to this, a large V wave causes the mean wedge pressure to overestimate the left ventricular end-diastolic pressure.[15] Remember, the mean wedge pressure reflects the entire cardiac cycle, while the left ventricular end diastolic pressure is a single time point measurement. For the best estimate of the left ventricular end diastolic (filling) pressure in the presence of a large V wave, measure the wedge pressure at a single time point (end diastole).[15] The end of the wedge pressure A wave (post A wave pressure) coincides with the end of left ventricular diastole. In the presence of a large V wave, measurement of the post A wave wedge pressure allows a reliable estimate of left ventricular filling pressure *(Figure 5.1)*.

For clinical purposes, the mean wedge pressure reflects the hydrostatic force in the pulmonary capillary bed. A large V wave will raise the mean wedge pressure and promote pulmonary edema formation. If the patient's primary problem is respiratory failure due to pulmonary congestion, then the effort should be directed at lowering the mean wedge pressure. On the other hand, if the patient's primary problem is a low cardiac output, attention should be directed at maintaining an adequate left ventricular filling pressure (post A wave pressure in the wedge waveform).

 ## Key Points: Acute Mitral Regurgitation & the V Wave

- Acute mitral regurgitation results in a large V wave in the wedge pressure waveform. This, in turn, significantly increases the mean wedge pressure.

- A large V wave is often observed in conditions other than acute mitral regurgitation.

- A large V wave is often transmitted retrograde to the pulmonary artery resulting in a bifid appearance to the pulmonary artery waveform.

- In the presence of a large V wave, the pulmonary artery diastolic pressure underestimates the mean wedge pressure.

- In the presence of a large V wave, the mean wedge pressure overestimates the left ventricular end diastolic pressure (filling pressure).

- The volume of mitral regurgitation cannot be measured with either the Fick or thermodilution cardiac output methods.

Chapter 5 References

1. Ronan JA, Steelman RB, DeLeon AC, Waters TJ, Percloff JK, Harvey WP. The clinical diagnosis of acute severe mitral insufficiency. *Am J Cardiol* 1971;27:284-290.

2. DePace NL, Nestico PF, Morganroth J. Acute severe mitral regurgitation: Pathophysiology, clinical recognition, and management. *Am J Med* 1985;78:293-306.

3. Braunwald E, Awe WC. The syndrome of severe mitral regurgitation with normal left atrial pressure. *Circulation* 1963; 27:29-35.

4. Levinson DC, Wilburne M, Meehan JP, Shubin H. Evidence for retrograde trans-pulmonary propagation of the V (or regurgitant) wave in mitral insufficiency. *Am J Cardiol* 1958; 2:159-169.

5. Grose R, Strain J, Cohen MV. Pulmonary arterial V waves in mitral regurgitation: Clinical and experimental observations. *Circulation* 1984;69:214-222.

6. Tatooles CJ, Gault JH, Mason DT, Ross J. Reflux of oxygenated blood into the pulmonary artery in severe mitral regurgitation. *Am Heart J* 1968;75:102-106.

7. Pichard AD, Kay R, Smith H, Rentrop P, Holt J, Gorlin R. Large V waves in the pulmonary wedge pressure tracing in the absence of mitral regurgitation. *Am J Cardiol* 1982; 50:1044-1050.

8. Fuchs RM, Henser RR, Yin FCP, Brinker JA. Limitations of pulmonary wedge V waves in diagnosing mitral regurgitation. *Am J Cardiol* 1982;49:849-854.

9. Bethen CF, Peter RH, Behar VS, Margolis JR, Kisslo JA, Kong Y. The hemodynamic simulation of mitral regurgitation in ventricular septal defect after myocardial infarction. *Cathet Cardiovasc Diagn* 1976; 2:97-104.

10. Yoran C, Yellin EL, Becker RM. Dynamic aspects of acute mitral regurgitation: Effects of ventricular volume, pressure, and contractility on the effective regurgitant orifice area. *Circulation* 1989; 60:170-176.

11. Brody W, Criley JM. Intermittent severe mitral regurgitation. Hemodynamic studies in a patient with recurrent acute left-sided heart failure. *N Engl J Med* 1970; 283:673-676.

12. Markiewicz W, Amikam S, Roguin N, Riss E. Changing haemodynamics in patient with papillary muscle dysfunction. *British Heart Journal* 1975;37:445-448.

13. Sharkey SW, Aberg NB. Hemodynamic evidence of painless myocardial ischemia with acute pulmonary edema in coronary disease. *Am Heart J* 1995;129:188-191.

14. Harshaw CW, Murro AB, McLaurin LP, Grossman W. Reduced systemic vascular resistance as therapy for severe mitral regurgitation. *Ann Intern Med* 1975; 83:312-316.

15. Haskell RJ, French WJ. Accuracy of left atrial and pulmonary artery wedge pressure in pure mitral regurgitation in predicting left ventricular end-diastolic pressure. *Am J Cardiol* 1988; 61:136-41.

CHAPTER **6**

TRICUSPID REGURGITATION

Tricuspid regurgitation is a chronic condition caused by right ventricular failure and dilatation.[1-3] The right ventricular failure can often be traced to long standing pulmonary artery hypertension.[4,5] Tricuspid regurgitation changes the right atrial pressure waveform, raises the right atrial mean pressure, and may invalidate the thermodilution method of measuring cardiac output *(Chapter 3)*. Furthermore, advancing the balloon-tipped catheter from the right atrium into the right ventricle is often challenging in these patients because of the regurgitant jet of blood. Fluoroscopy may be necessary to properly position the catheter when tricuspid regurgitation is severe.

Right Atrial Pressure

The classic pressure waveform of tricuspid regurgitation is a large broad C-V wave followed by a steep Y descent.[6-8] The tricuspid valve begins to leak with the onset of right ventricular systole. The onset of right ventricular systole is marked by the C wave in the right atrial pressure waveform. As the tricuspid regurgitation progresses during ventricular systole the right atrial pressure progressively rises. The X' descent is therefore attenuated or obliterated. The result is a fusion of the C and V waves into a

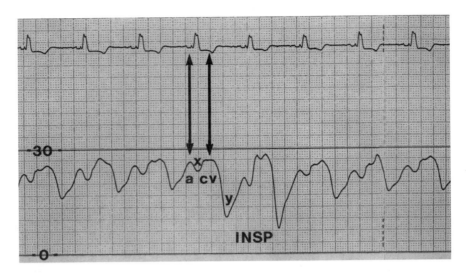

Figure 6.1 Right atrial pressure waveform from a patient with severe tricuspid regurgitation after long standing pulmonary hypertension. The rhythm is sinus. The mean right atrial pressure is elevated at 22 mmHg. The A wave (**a**) and the X descent (**x**) are normal. The X′ descent is obliterated by the tricuspid regurgitation. The result is a broad positive C-V wave (**cv**) that is higher than the A wave. Note that inspiration (**INSP**) magnifies the peak of the C-V wave and the nadir of the Y descent (**y**). As a result, the mean right atrial pressure shows little respiratory variation. Scale = 0-30 mmHg; Paper speed = 25 mm/sec.

single broad positive wave (the so called C-V wave) *(Figure 6.1)*. As the degree of tricuspid regurgitation increases, the right atrial C-V wave becomes more accentuated.[9] The C-V wave of tricuspid regurgitation is never as striking as the C-V wave of acute mitral regurgitation because tricuspid regurgitation is a chronic condition that develops gradually. Furthermore, the left ventricle usually generates a much higher systolic pressure than does the right ventricle.

The Y descent is the dominant feature of the right atrial pressure waveform with significant tricuspid regurgitation *(Figure 6.1)*. The Y descent is exaggerated because the high pressure within the right atrium is suddenly relieved as the tricuspid valve opens and the right atrial blood volume is delivered to the right ventricle at the beginning of diastole. This striking Y descent is readily observed by examining the jugular veins of these patients. During inspiration the C-V wave is augmented and the Y descent becomes more pronounced *(Figure 6.1)*. As a result, the mean right atrial pressure remains constant or may even rise (Kussmaul's sign).[10]

In patients with sinus rhythm, an A wave followed by a small X descent is present in the right atrial pressure waveform *(Figure 6.1)*. The A wave is usually smaller than the C-V wave.

During atrial fibrillation, the absent A wave causes the right atrial pressure waveform to resemble that seen with tricuspid regurgitation even when the tricuspid valve is competent.[11,12] Use caution when interpreting the right atrial pressure waveform in the presence of atrial fibrillation *(Chapter 4)*.

The right atrial pressure waveform of tricuspid regurgitation will be modified by the size and distensibility of the right atrium. When the right atrium is very dilated and compliant, the characteristic C-V wave and steep Y descent may be attenuated or even absent despite severe tricuspid regurgitation[7,11] *(Figure 6.2)*. In this setting, the characteristic thermodilution cardiac output curve may provide a helpful clue to the presence of significant tricuspid regurgitation *(Chapter 3)*. Doppler echocardiography is a particularly useful way to evaluate the severity of tricuspid regurgitation.

With tricuspid regurgitation, the mean right atrial pressure is elevated. In addition, the ratio of right atrial/wedge pressure increases. The right atrial pressure may equal or exceed the wedge pressure, especially when the tricuspid regurgitation occurs in the absence of left heart disease. When the right atrial pressure exceeds the wedge pressure, right to left shunting or paradoxical embolization can occur through a patent foramen ovale.[13,14] This shunt can be visualized with two-dimensional echocardiography when contrast is injected into the venous circulation.[15]

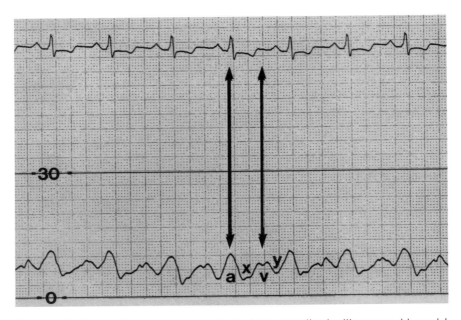

Figure 6.2 Right atrial pressure waveform from a patient with severe tricuspid regurgitation from chronic pulmonary hypertension due to cirrhosis of the liver. The mean right atrial pressure is minimally elevated at 6 mmHg. The A wave (**a**) is the dominant feature of the tracing. The C wave (**c**) is not visible. The diagnosis of tricuspid regurgitation cannot be made from this pressure tracing. Two-dimensional echocardiography revealed severe tricuspid regurgitation and marked right atrial enlargement. The thermodilution cardiac output curve was typical of severe tricuspid regurgitation. Scale = 0-30 mmHg; Paper speed = 25 mm/sec.

Pulmonary Artery Pressure

Pulmonary hypertension is the rule and may be severe. An important exception to this rule can be observed with right ventricular infarction where right ventricular dilation is caused by ischemic injury and not pulmonary hypertension. When present, pulmonary hypertension may be caused by either left heart disease or primary pulmonary disease. The wedge pressure may be normal or elevated depending on whether left heart disease is present.

Key Points: Tricuspid Regurgitation

- The right atrial pressure is elevated with a broad positive C-V wave. The X′ descent is attenuated or absent while the Y descent is prominent.

- Kussmaul's sign may be present.

- The thermodilution cardiac output method is often inaccurate with significant tricuspid regurgitation.

- The right atrial pressure may equal or exceed the wedge pressure (left atrial pressure) setting the stage for right to left shunting and paradoxical embolization.

Chapter 6 References

1. Mikami T, Kudo T, Sakurai N, Sakamoto S, Tanabe Y, Yasuda H. Mechanisms for development of functional tricuspid regurgitation determined by pulsed Doppler and two-dimensional echocardiography. *Am J Cardiol* 1984; 53:160-163.

2. Come PC and Riley MF. Tricuspid annular dilatation and failure of tricuspid leaflet coaptation in patients with tricuspid regurgitation. *Am J Cardiol* 1985; 55:599-601.

3. Waller BF, Moriarity AT, Eble JN, Davey DM, Hawley DA, Pless JE. Etiology of pure tricuspid regurgitation based on annular circumference and leaflet area: Analysis of 45 necropsy patients with clinical and morphologic evidence of pure tricuspid regurgitation. *J Am Coll Cardiol* 1986; 7:1063-1074.

4. Ockene IS. Tricuspid valve disease. In: Dalen JE, Alpert JS, editors. *Valvular Heart Disease.* Boston: Little, Brown, 1981: 281-328.

5. Salazar E, Levine HD. Rheumatic tricuspid regurgitation: The clinical spectrum. *Am J Med* 1962; 33:111-129.

6. Messer AL, Hurst JW, Rappaport MB, Sprague HB. A study of the venous pulse in tricuspid valve disease. *Circulation* 1950; 1:388-393.

7. Rubeiz GA, Nassar ME, Dagher IK. Study of the right atrial pressure pulse in functional tricuspid regurgitation and normal sinus rhythm. *Circulation* 1964; 30:190-193.

8. Cha SD, Rashmikant SD, Gooch AS, Maranhao V, Goldberg H. Diagnosis of severe tricuspid regurgitation. *Chest* 1982; 82:726-731.

9. Constant J. *Bedside Cardiology,* 3rd ed. Boston: Little, Brown, 1985: 95, 105, 108.

10. Lingamneni R, Cha SD, Maranhao V, Gooch AS, Goldberg H. Tricuspid regurgitation: Clinical and angiographic assessment. *Cathet Cardiovasc Diagn* 1979; 5:7-17.

11. Cairns KB, Kloster FE, Bristow JD, Lees MH, Griswold HE. Problems in the hemodynamic diagnosis of tricuspid insufficiency. *Am Heart J* 1968;75:173-179.

12. Gould L, Weber D, Schaffer AI, O'Connor RA. Does atrial fibrillation lead to tricuspid insufficiency? *Am J Cardiol* 1965; 6:189-194.

13. Hagen PT, Scholz DG, Edwards WD. Incidence and size of patent foramen ovale during the first 10 decades of life: An autopsy study of 965 normal hearts. *Mayo Clin Proc* 1984; 59:17-20.

14. Gazzaniga AB, Dalen JE. Paradoxical embolism: Its pathophysiology and clinical recognition. *Ann Surg* 1970; 171:137-142.

15. Berger BC, Walinsky P, Carey P. Primary pulmonary hypertension: M-mode and two-dimensional echocardiographic findings. *Cathet Cardiovasc Diagn* 1983, 9:187-195.

ACUTE LEFT VENTRICULAR INFARCTION

T he hemodynamic consequences of an acute myocardial infarction encompass the entire spectrum. The size and location of the infarction, the mitral valve function, the heart rate and rhythm, and the pre-existing left ventricular function are all variables which influence the hemodynamic measurements. Right ventricular infarction complicating an inferior left ventricular infarction is associated with unique hemodynamic findings and is discussed in Chapter 8. The hemodynamic abnormalities of acute left ventricular infarction are confined largely to the wedge pressure, the cardiac index, and the arterial blood pressure.

Physiologic Effects of Left Ventricular Infarction

The hallmark of acute infarction is a sudden loss of regional myocardial systolic and diastolic function. This regional contractile dysfunction is compensated by enhanced contraction of available normal myocardium. In the 1970's, investigators reported the relation between infarct size and parameters of left ventricular function.[1] Abnormal left ventricular compliance can be measured with an infarction involving only 8% of the left ventricle. When the infarction exceeds 10% of the left ventricle, the ejection fraction

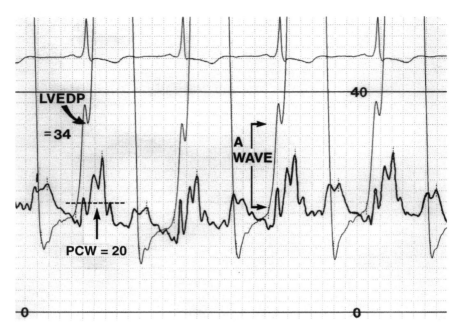

Figure 7.1 Noncompliant left ventricle disrupting the relationship of mean wedge pressure to left ventricular end diastolic pressure (**LVEDP**). Recordings made in the Catheterization Lab from a patient with acute myocardial infarction. The LVEDP is markedly elevated at 34 mmHg. The mean wedge pressure (**PCW**) of 20 mmHg seriously underestimates the LVEDP because of a very large **A wave**. The A wave amplitude is nearly 16 mmHg. Scale = 0-40 mmHg; Paper speed = 50 mm/sec.

is reduced; with 15% infarction, the left ventricular end-diastolic pressure is increased. When the infarct exceeds 25% of the left ventricle, clinically evident congestive heart failure occurs. Cardiogenic shock, the most extreme form of heart failure, appears when acute infarction involves 40% or more of the left ventricle.

The hemodynamic consequences of an acute left ventricular infarction are confined mainly to a variable increase in the left ventricular end-diastolic pressure and a variable decrease in the stroke volume. Acute infarction alters left ventricular compliance causing a shift in the Frank-Starling relationship. Therefore, patients with acute myocardial infarction will often require a higher than normal left ventricular end-diastolic pressure to achieve optimal stroke volume and cardiac output.[2] In patients with acute infarction, optimal left ventricular stroke volume occurs with a left ventricular end-diastolic pressure of 20-25 mmHg.[2]

The normal close correlation between the mean wedge pressure and the left ventricular end-diastolic pressure is disrupted by an acute myocardial infarction.[3,4] The left atrial contribution to the left ventricular end-diastolic pressure ("booster pump" action) is increased.[5,6] In normal hearts, left atrial systole raises the left ventricular diastolic pressure by only 1-2 mmHg.[5,6] With acute infarction, left atrial contraction augments the left ventricular diastolic pressure by an average of 8 mmHg.[3,4] This several fold increase in the A wave (atrial systole) is caused by reduced left ventricular compliance. The mean wedge pressure significantly underestimates the left ventricular end-diastolic pressure (on average by 8-10 mmHg) because of the large A wave (*Figure 7.1*). This fact explains the important observation that the optimal mean wedge pressure for patients with an acute myocardial infarction is 14-18 mmHg which corresponds to a left ventricular end-diastolic pressure of 20-25 mmHg (*Figure 7.2*).[7] In patients with a very noncompliant infarction (and a very large A wave), the optimal mean wedge pressure may be below 15 mmHg (*Figure 7.3*). Thus the ideal mean wedge pressure during an acute myocardial infarction varies with the individual. In critically ill patients, the effect of increasing or decreasing the mean wedge pressure should be carefully assessed by measuring the response of the cardiac output and the stroke volume. As a rule, there is little to gain by increasing the mean wedge pressure above 18-20 mmHg.[7]

Hemodynamic Spectrum of Acute Myocardial Infarction

Careful study of consecutive patients with an acute myocardial infarction has shown that the mean wedge pressure exceeds 18 mmHg in 50% of patients.[8,9] The cardiac index is depressed (< 2.5

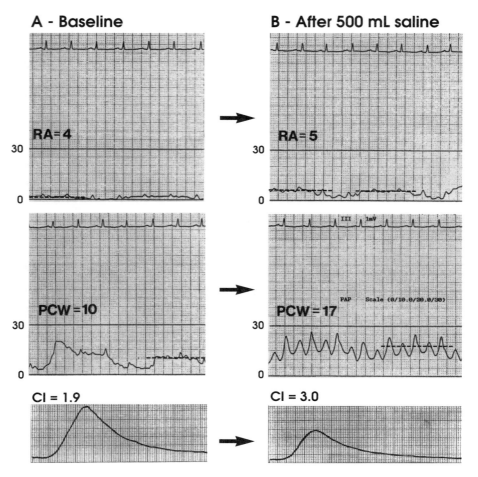

Figure 7.2 Optimal wedge pressure in acute myocardial infarction. Recording of right atrial pressure (**RA**), wedge pressure (**PCW**), and cardiac index (**CI**) from a patient with acute anterior myocardial infarction and clinical low output state. **Panel A:** At baseline (left), the cardiac index is significantly reduced at 1.9 L/min/m^2 with normal right atrial and wedge pressures. **Panel B:** (right) after 500 mL saline bolus, the wedge pressure increases to 17 mmHg (near optimum for an acute infarction) with a dramatic improvement in the cardiac index to 3.0 L/min/m^2. The stroke volume index improved from 18 mL/beat/m^2 to 30 mL/beat/m^2. Note that the saline bolus had little effect on the right atrial pressure in this patient with acute infarction of the left ventricle. Note also that the A and V waves are easily visible in the wedge tracing after the volume challenge because the left atrial pressure now exceeds the alveolar pressure (allowing retrograde waveform transmission).
Scale = 0-30 mmHg; Paper speed = 25 mm/sec.

Figure 7.3 Acute anterior infarction with a non-compliant left ventricle. Recordings made in the Catheterization Lab.
Panel A: At baseline, the wedge (**PCW**) pressure is 11-12 mmHg and the cardiac index (**CI**) is 2.3 L/min/m^2.

A - Baseline

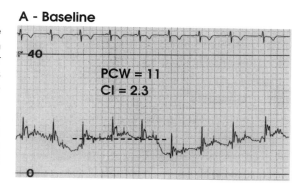

PCW = 11
CI = 2.3

Panel B: At baseline, the left ventricular end-diastolic pressure (**LVEDP**) is 31 mmHg; the PCW therefore underestimates the LVEDP by 21 mmHg. This is caused by the presence of a large
A Wave (16 mmHg amplitude) in the left ventricular pressure tracing.

B - Baseline

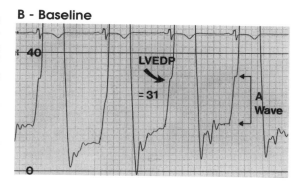

LVEDP
= 31

A Wave

Panel C: The patient was given 500 mL of saline because of hypotension. The wedge pressure increased to 21 mmHg but the cardiac index did not improve because the LVEDP was adequate before the volume challenge. In this patient, recording the left ventricular pressure in the Catheterization Lab

C - After 500 mL saline

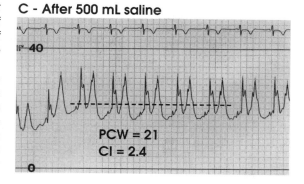

PCW = 21
CI = 2.4

provided the explanation for the failure of the cardiac index to rise after a volume challenge. Scale = 0-40 mmHg; Paper speed = 25 mm/sec (Panels A & C) and 50 mm/sec (Panel B).

L/min/m^2) in 50% of patients.[8,9] Forrester, Swan and colleagues described the correlation of hemodynamic measurements with hospital mortality in patients with acute myocardial infarction.[8,9] Patients can be triaged into one of four hemodynamic subsets based on measurement of the mean wedge pressure and the cardiac index (*Table 7.1*). A depressed cardiac index confers a mortality increase of 5 to 15 fold depending on whether or not the wedge pressure is also increased.[8-10] Likewise, an increased wedge pressure raises the mortality by 2 to 15 fold depending on whether or not the cardiac index is also decreased.[8-10] It is important to note that these observations were made prior to the era of emergency reperfusion therapy for acute myocardial infarction.

Hemodynamic & Clinical Correlates

Wedge Pressure & Pulmonary Congestion

As the left ventricular end-diastolic pressure increases with acute myocardial infarction, so does the mean wedge pressure. The increased hydrostatic pressure promotes pulmonary congestion and ultimately pulmonary edema. Clinically, this is manifest as dyspnea and respiratory failure. As a rule, the degree of elevation of the mean wedge pressure correlates with the degree of pulmonary congestion as follows:[10,11]

Mean Wedge Pressure	Degree of Pulmonary Congestion
18 - 20 mmHg	Onset of pulmonary congestion
21 - 25 mmHg	Moderate congestion
26 - 30 mmHg	Severe congestion
> 30 mmHg	Acute pulmonary edema

Pulmonary congestion is recognized clinically using the stethoscope (presence of post-tussive rales) or based on the chest x-ray findings. The predictive accuracy of the clinical evaluation for the presence of a mean wedge pressure > 18 mmHg is 85%.[8,9] Failure to recognize a mean wedge pressure > 18 mmHg occurs in

Table 7.1 Hemodynamic Subsets in Acute Myocardial Infarction				
Subset	Wedge Pressure > 18 mmHg	Cardiac Index < 2.2 L/min/m²	Observed Frequency	Hospital Mortality
I	No	No	31%	3%
II	Yes	No	17%	9%
III	No	Yes	17%	23%
IV	Yes	Yes	35%	51%

Adapted from Forrester JS, et al. Medical therapy of acute myocardial infarction by application of hemodynamic subsets. *N Engl J Med* 1976;295:1361.

15% of patients.[8,9]   Discrepancies between the clinical findings of pulmonary congestion and the wedge pressure measurement have several explanations. The "phase-lag" phenomenon is particularly common; improvement in the physical examination and x-ray findings often lags behind improvement in the mean wedge pressure (by hours or even days).[12] Another source of confusion is the nonspecific nature of pulmonary rales. Many patients with acute myocardial infarction have coexisting chronic lung disease. In these patients, rales may be a marker for the presence of intrinsic lung disease and not an elevated mean wedge pressure. Finally, patients with pre-existing heart disease may tolerate a higher mean wedge pressure without developing pulmonary congestion. Chronic heart failure promotes physical changes in the pulmonary vasculature together with improved lymphatic drainage, both of which work to mask the presence of an elevated wedge pressure.[8,9]

Cardiac Index & Tissue Perfusion

A sudden decrease in the cardiac index is clinically manifest as decreased perfusion of the skin (cold, clammy), kidneys (oliguria), and brain (anxiety, lethargy). The degree of depression of the cardiac index corresponds to the severity of tissue hypoperfusion as follows.[10]

Cardiac Index	Severity of Tissue Hypoperfusion
2.5-3.5 L/min/m^2	Normal range
2.0-2.2 L/min/m^2	Onset of peripheral hypoperfusion
1.8-2.0 L/min/m^2	Onset of cardiogenic shock

The predictive accuracy of the clinical examination for detecting the presence of a cardiac index less than 2.2 L/min/m^2 is 81%.[8,9] The major limitation of the clinical evaluation is the failure to diagnose a depressed cardiac index in 14% of patients.[8,9]   The clinical-hemodynamic correlations described above apply to patients with an acute myocardial infarction. Patients with a chronically reduced cardiac index may not exhibit any of these findings. Long-term adaptations such as a shift in the oxyhemoglobin dissociation curve may allow adequate tissue oxygenation despite a serious reduction in the cardiac index.

Arterial Blood Pressure

The arterial blood pressure is normal in the majority of patients with acute myocardial infarction.[1,13] It is common to observe moderate hypertension (> 160/90 mmHg) even in previously normotensive patients due to the sympathetic discharge accompanying myocardial infarction.[1] The arterial pressure rarely exceeds 200/110 mmHg.[1] Hypotension (< 90 mmHg systolic) does not always signify the presence of cardiogenic shock. Activation of the Bezold-Jarisch reflex may result in profound peripheral vasodilation and hypotension. Stimulation of this reflex is more common in patients with acute inferior infarction.[14,15] The Bezold-Jarisch reflex can also be stimulated by reperfusion and by administration of nitroglycerin[16,17] (*Figure 7.4*). Patients with hypotension mediated by high vagal tone usually appear warm and well perfused. The vagus nerve action also promotes bradycardia in these patients.

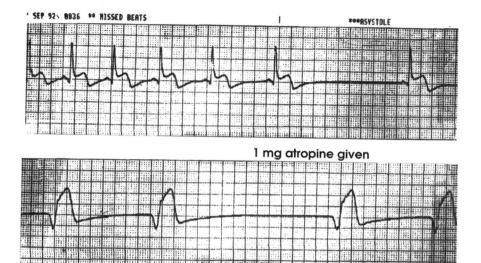

Figure 7.4 Lead III rhythm strip demonstrates activation of the Bezold-Jarisch reflex by nitroglycerin. The patient has an acute inferior infarction. At baseline (08:36) sinus rhythm is present with ST-segment elevation. Administration of intravenous nitroglycerin resulted in profound sinus bradycardia and hypotension. This episode resolved quickly with administration of atropine and discontinuation of the nitroglycerin.

Mechanical Complications of Acute Myocardial Infarction

Cardiogenic Shock

Cardiogenic shock is the most feared consequence of acute myocardial infarction. It carries a mortality exceeding 70% and is the leading cause of hospital death in patients with an acute myocardial infarction.[18-21] Patients who die from cardiogenic shock have pathologic evidence for infarction involving 40% or more of the left ventricular myocardium.[22]

Cardiogenic shock is a clinical diagnosis defined by the triad of:[18]

- Hypotension: systolic blood pressure ≤ 90 mmHg (prior to inotropic or intraaortic balloon pump support)
- Poor tissue perfusion
- Pulmonary congestion

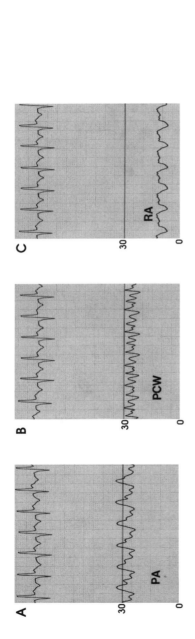

Figure 7.5   (Panels A-D) Intracardiac pressure recordings from a patient with an acute anterior myocardial infarction, right bundle branch block, and cardiogenic shock. Sinus tachycardia (129 beats/min) is present. **Panel A:** Modest pulmonary artery (**PA**) hypertension (33/24 mmHg) is present. The pulmonary artery pulse pressure is reduced (9 mmHg) because of reduced stroke volume.

Panel B: The mean pulmonary capillary wedge pressure (**PCW**) is elevated at 25 mmHg. Pulmonary edema was present on chest x-ray. The mean wedge pressure correlates well with the pulmonary artery diastolic pressure.

Panel C: The mean right atrial pressure (**RA**) is elevated at 11 mmHg. The ratio of right atrial pressure to wedge pressure is 0.4. The A wave and V wave have begun to merge because of sinus tachycardia. As a result, the y descent is blunted. **Panel D:** Thermodilution cardiac output curve recorded from this patient. The cardiac index is significantly reduced at 1.7 liters/min/m² (body surface area = 1.8 m²). The stroke volume is markedly reduced at 23 mL/beat. The cardiac output is maintained at the level of 3.0 liters/min by sinus tachycardia together with intravenous dopamine and an intraaortic balloon pump. Without intraaortic balloon pump support, the cardiac output and stroke volume were 2.6 liters/minute and 20 mL/beat respectively.

Patients with cardiogenic shock have a reduced cardiac index combined with an elevated wedge pressure corresponding to hemodynamic subset IV in the Forrester Classification Scheme *(Table 7.1)*.

Intracardiac Pressures in Cardiogenic Shock

The right atrial, pulmonary artery and wedge pressures are all elevated. The degree of intracardiac pressure elevation is not nearly as striking as that observed in patients with chronic congestive heart failure *(Chapter 10)*. Typical intracardiac pressures observed in patients with cardiogenic shock include: mean right atrial pressure of 12-16 mmHg; pulmonary artery systolic pressure of 35-45 mmHg; pulmonary artery diastolic pressure of 18-30 mmHg; and mean wedge pressure of 18-30 mmHg[23-25] *(Figure 7.5)*.

With cardiogenic shock, the ratio of the mean right atrial pressure to the mean wedge pressure is usually 0.5.[23-25] Of course, this ratio will be closer to 1.0 when cardiogenic shock complicates right ventricular infarction *(Chapter 8)*. The right atrial pressure waveform may demonstrate summation of the A and V waves because of the presence of pronounced sinus tachycardia *(Figure 7.5, Panel C)*.

The mean wedge pressure is usually elevated to a level that causes clinical pulmonary congestion or overt pulmonary edema.[20, 23-25] The diagnosis of cardiogenic shock requires that the patient has received adequate volume expansion so that the mean wedge pressure at least exceeds 12 mmHg.[18] Remember, optimal cardiac performance during acute myocardial infarction occurs with a mean wedge pressure of 14-18 mmHg[7] *(Figure 7.6)*. Maneuvers that increase the mean wedge pressure beyond this range may cause cardiac performance to worsen.[7] The A and V waves are usually of similar magnitude *(Figure 7.5, Panel B)*. A large V wave suggests the presence of significant acute mitral regurgitation *(Chapter 5)*.

While the pulmonary artery systolic and diastolic pressures are both elevated, the pulse pressure may be narrow reflecting a decrease in the stroke volume *(Figure 7.5, Panel A)*.[23-25] The close correlation between the pulmonary artery diastolic pressure and the mean wedge pressure is generally preserved in these patients[26] *(Figure 7.5, Panel A & B)*. In an occasional patient, the pulmonary artery diastolic pressure is significantly greater than the mean wedge pressure because of an increased pulmonary vascular resistance.[26]

Cardiac Index in Cardiogenic Shock

Clinical cardiogenic shock is associated with a cardiac index ≤ 1.8 liters/min/m^2. [8,9,26] The cardiac index is critically dependent on the heart rate. Sinus tachycardia often compensates for a striking decrease in the stroke volume *(Figure 7.5, Panel D)*. It is crucial to calculate the stroke volume since a change in the cardiac index may be caused simply by a change in the heart rate and not the intrinsic cardiac performance. It is also important to consider that the cardiac index measurement will be influenced by the use of inotropic drugs and/or intraaortic balloon pump support. Each cardiac index measurement should therefore include documentation of the heart rate, the dose of inotropic drugs, and the level of intraaortic balloon pump support.

Arterial Blood Pressure in Cardiogenic Shock

The cuff blood pressure is notoriously inaccurate in patients with cardiogenic shock.[18] Cuff pressures can underestimate the actual intraarterial pressure by as much as 160 mmHg.[27] Intraarterial pressure measurement is mandatory. Moderate to severe systolic hypotension ≤ 90 mmHg is the rule.[26] The aortic pulse pressure may be reduced as a consequence of a low left ventricular stroke volume.

Intraaortic Balloon Pump in Cardiogenic Shock

An intraaortic balloon pump is often used to support the circulation in patients with cardiogenic shock.[28] The balloon pump inflation/deflation cycle occurs during diastole and produces a

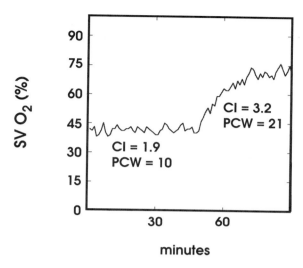

Figure 7.6 Continuous recording of mixed venous oxygen saturation (**SV O$_2$**) from a patient with acute anterior myocardial infarction and shock. At baseline, the cardiac index (**CI**) was 1.9 L/min/m^2 and the wedge pressure (**PCW**) was 10 mmHg. The mixed venous saturation at this point was 40-45%. After volume expansion with blood and albumen, the cardiac index rose to 3.2 L/min/m^2. The rapid rise of the mixed venous saturation to 70-75% reflects the improved cardiac index. In this patient, the change in the mixed venous oxygen saturation provided nearly instant confirmation that volume expansion was beneficial.

predictable effect on the arterial pressure, the mean wedge pressure, and the stroke volume. The intraaortic balloon pump is programmed to inflate at the moment of aortic valve closure (dicrotic notch) and to deflate prior to the onset of aortic ejection (aortic pressure upstroke *Figure 7.7*). A peripheral arterial catheter cannot be used to precisely coordinate the balloon pump cycle because of the time required for the pressure waveform to travel from the aortic valve to the extremities. A proximal aortic pressure recording is essential.

Balloon pump inflation causes a sudden augmentation of the early aortic diastolic blood pressure (*Figure 7.7*). This promotes tissue perfusion and increases the diastolic coronary artery blood flow velocity.[29] Balloon pump deflation lowers the aortic end-

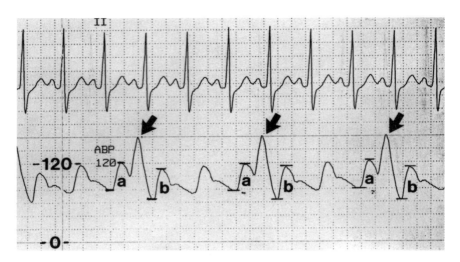

Figure 7.7 Arterial blood pressure recording demonstrating the effects of an intraaortic balloon pump (IABP) on the aortic pressure waveform. The IABP inflation/deflation (**arrows**) occurs every third beat (1:3). Inflation occurs at aortic valve closure (dicrotic notch). Deflation occurs before the onset of ejection of the next beat. The IABP inflation augments the early diastolic pressure of beat "**a**". Note that IABP deflation lowers the aortic end-diastolic pressure so that beat "**b**" begins ejection against a lower "afterload." The stroke volume of beat "b" is therefore improved. This results in a higher aortic pulse pressure (compare the pulse pressure of beat "a" with that of beat "b"). Scale = 0-120 mmHg; Paper speed = 25 mm/sec.

diastolic pressure and provides a mechanical advantage (decreased afterload) for the next left ventricular ejection *(Figure 7.7)*. As a result, the stroke volume of the damaged left ventricle rises and contributes to an improved cardiac output *(Figure 7.8)*. The mean wedge pressure may also decline because of the improved left ventricular ejection *(Figure 7.9)*. This is especially true when significant mitral valve regurgitation is present.

Mitral Regurgitation & Pericardial Tamponade
These complications of an acute myocardial infarction are uncommon especially since the advent of reperfusion therapy. Acute severe mitral regurgitation is the result of infarction of one of the papillary muscles and adjacent ventricular myocardium.

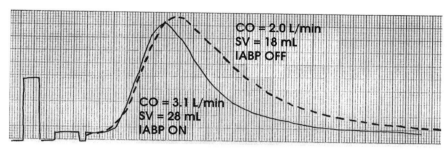

Figure 7.8 Effect of intraaortic balloon pump (IABP) support on the cardiac output (**CO** liters/min) and stroke volume (**SV**, mL per beat) in a patient with cardiogenic shock. The thermodilution cardiac output curve recorded with the IABP on (**solid line**) is superimposed with the cardiac output curve recorded with the IABP off (**dashed line**). The improved cardiac output is due solely to an improved stroke volume.

The hemodynamic consequences of acute mitral regurgitation are discussed in Chapter 5. Cardiac tamponade is the result of post-infarction pericarditis or sub-acute rupture of the left ventricular free wall.[30] The hemodynamic findings of cardiac tamponade are discussed in Chapter 11.

Ventricular Septal Rupture

Ventricular septal rupture can occur as a consequence of either anterior or inferior myocardial infarction. The result is a ventricular septal defect with a left to right shunt and a pulmonary-to-systemic blood flow ratio usually greater than 2:1.[31] The diagnosis of an acute left-to-right shunt can be confirmed by demonstrating a significant increase (10 percent or more) in the oxygen saturation between the right atrium and the pulmonary artery[32,33] (*Table 7.2*). The right atrial oxygen saturation must be interpreted carefully; this chamber receives blood from the inferior vena cava, the superior vena cava, and the coronary sinus. The right atrial oxygen saturation can be artificially decreased if the proximal catheter lumen is adjacent to the coronary sinus. On the other hand, the right atrial oxygen saturation can be artificially increased if significant tricuspid regurgitation further complicates

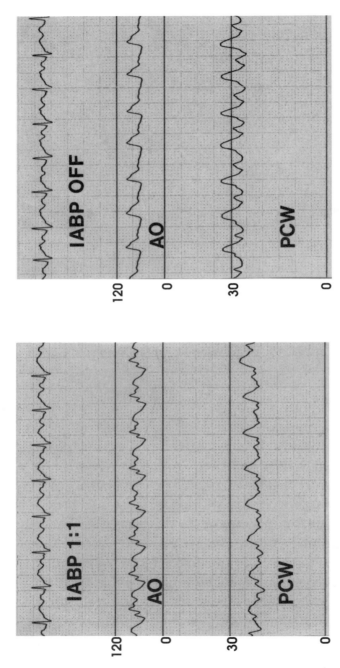

Figure 7.9 Effect of intraaortic balloon pump (**IABP**) support on the pulmonary capillary wedge (**PCW**) pressure in a patient with cardiogenic shock. **Left Panel:** IABP support is 1:1. The diastolic augmentation appears blunted because the aortic pressure (**AO**) recording was made from a peripheral femoral arterial line. The mean PCW is 23 mmHg. **Right Panel:** IABP has been discontinued for 15 seconds. The diastolic augmentation is now absent on the aortic pressure recording. The mean pulmonary capillary wedge pressure has abruptly risen to 29 mmHg. Note that the wedge pressure A and V waves are transmitted more effectively at the higher wedge pressure. Scale = 0-120 mmHg (AO) and 0-30 mmHg (PCW). Paper speed = 25 mm/sec.

the ventricular septal rupture. Oxygenated blood is shunted across the septal defect into the right ventricle and then refluxes across the tricuspid valve into the right atrium. This unusual scenario is most likely to occur when septal rupture complicates acute inferior myocardial infarction with concomitant right ventricular infarction and tricuspid papillary muscle dysfunction.

With an acute ventricular septal defect, the mean right atrial, wedge, and pulmonary artery pressures are all significantly elevated[31,34] *(Table 7.2)*. A large V wave is often present in the wedge pressure tracing.[35,36] Acute ventricular septal defect and acute mitral regurgitation share many clinical and hemodynamic features. Whenever a patient with acute myocardial infarction develops heart failure, a systolic murmur, and a large V wave in the wedge pressure waveform, the astute clinician should consider both ventricular septal rupture and severe mitral regurgitation. With acute septal rupture, the systemic blood flow averages only one-half to one-fourth of the thermodilution determined cardiac output. Remember, the thermodilution method measures the pulmonary blood flow (right-sided cardiac output). Thus, a "normal" thermodilution measured cardiac output in a patient with acute septal rupture usually reflects a severe reduction in systemic blood flow.

Table 7.2 Hemodynamic Parameters and Oxygen Saturations in a Patient with Acute Ventricular Septal Defect	
Right atrial pressure	18 mmHg
Pulmonary artery pressure	54/17 mmHg
Pulmonary capillary wedge pressure	22 mmHg
Cardiac output (thermodilution)	4.2 liters/minute
Right atrial oxygen saturation	49%
Pulmonary artery oxygen saturation	61%

Role of Hemodynamic Monitoring in Guiding Treatment

Most patients with acute myocardial infarction do not require invasive monitoring because of the close correlation between clinical and hemodynamic findings. Bedside hemodynamic monitoring is reserved for the more seriously ill patient. The goal of therapy is to optimize the wedge pressure, the cardiac index, and the blood pressure to ensure survival of the patient. As such, therapy should not be based solely on the hemodynamic measurements; the patient's clinical status must be integrated with the hemodynamic findings. For example, efforts to raise a depressed cardiac index are most important when there is clinical evidence of poor peripheral perfusion. Likewise, measures to lower an increased wedge pressure are most important when pulmonary edema is present. The principles of effective treatment include:

- Assess the heart rate and rhythm. Sinus rhythm is most efficient.

- Maintain an optimal wedge pressure. A wedge pressure above 20 mmHg is rarely beneficial and may result in pulmonary congestion.

- Consider early use of reperfusion therapy. There is a lag between successful reperfusion and hemodynamic benefit because of myocardial stunning.

- Diuretic drugs are effective in lowering an elevated wedge pressure.

- Vasodilator drugs are most effective in patients with both elevated wedge pressure and reduced cardiac index, provided the arterial blood pressure is maintained.

- Inotropic drugs are useful in patients with reduced blood pressure and reduced cardiac index. These drugs may aggravate myocardial ischemia due to an increased heart rate and contractility. Consider an intraaortic balloon pump first.

- An intraaortic balloon pump is very effective for patients with reduced blood pressure and reduced cardiac index. An added benefit is the relief of residual myocardial ischemia.

The ideal heart rate for patients with acute myocardial infarction is highly individual. Sinus tachycardia may be a response to pain and catecholamine release, in which case administration of a beta blocker is indicated. In contrast, sinus tachycardia may be responsible for maintaining an adequate cardiac index; in this situation administration of a beta blocker would be harmful. Persistent bradycardia below 50 beats/min is usually not well tolerated. Treatment usually requires a pacemaker. Most temporary pacemakers are designed for ventricular pacing. Selecting the optimal ventricular rate can be performed by increasing the rate in increments of 10 beats/min beginning with 60 beats/min and measuring the effect on the cardiac index and blood pressure *(Figure 7.10)*. Ventricular pacemakers cause AV dissociation. The loss of AV synchrony can be clinically important in some patients. Patients with right ventricular infarction are particularly sensitive to the loss of AV synchrony *(Chapter 8)*. Temporary pacemakers which offer AV sequential pacing are available but difficult to use.

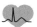 Key Points: Acute Left Ventricular Infarction

- The hemodynamic effects of acute left ventricular infarction involve the mean wedge pressure, the cardiac index, and the arterial blood pressure.

- There is very good correlation between hemodynamic measurements and clinical findings; both can be used to predict hospital mortality.

- The optimal mean wedge pressure for acute myocardial infarction is 15-20 mmHg.

Pacing at 60 beats/min

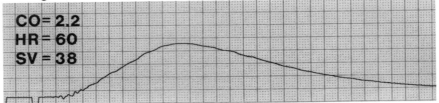

Pacing at 89 beats/min

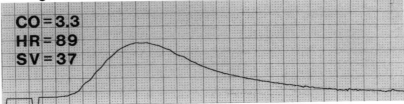

Figure 7.10 Effect of increasing heart rate on the cardiac output. The patient has an acute inferior infarction with complete heart block and a temporary ventricular pacemaker. At baseline (top), the cardiac output (**CO**) is 2.2 L/min at a heart rate (**HR**) of 60 beats/min. The effects of a higher heart rate were assessed because of oliguria and hypotension. An increase in the heart rate of 30 beats/min improved the cardiac output resulting in an increased blood pressure and improved urine flow. Note that the stroke volume (**SV**) is fixed. The improved cardiac output is due solely to the increased heart rate.

- Pulmonary edema appears when the mean wedge pressure exceeds 25-30 mmHg.

- The mean wedge pressure often underestimates the left ventricular end-diastolic pressure because of abnormal left ventricular compliance.

- Clinical cardiogenic shock is associated with an elevated mean wedge pressure (> 18 mmHg), a reduced cardiac index (< 2.2 L/min/m^2), and arterial hypotension (systolic ≤ 90 mmHg).

- Complications of acute myocardial infarction include septal rupture, mitral regurgitation, and pericardial tamponade. Each has unique hemodynamic features.

Chapter 7 References

1. Pasternak RC, Braunwald E, Sobel BE. Acute myocardial infarction. In: Braunwald E, ed. *Heart Disease: A Textbook of Cardiovascular Medicine*. Philadelphia: W.B. Saunders Co. 1988;1230.

2. Russell RO, Rackley CE, Pombo J, Hunt D, Potanin C, Dodge HT. Effects of increasing left ventricular filling pressure in patients with acute myocardial infarction. *J Clin Invest* 1970; 49:1539-1550.

3. Rahimtoola SH, Loeb HS, Ehsani A, Sinno MZ, Chuquimia R, Lal R, Rosen KM, Gunnar RM. Relationship of pulmonary artery to left ventricular diastolic pressures in acute myocardial infarction. *Circulation* 1972;46:283-290.

4. Broder MI, Cohn JN. Evolution of abnormalities in left ventricular function after acute myocardial infarction. *Circulation* 1972;46:731-743.

5. Braunwald E, Brockenbrough E, Frahm CJ, Ross JR. Left atrial and left ventricular pressures in subjects without cardiovascular disease: Observations in eighteen patients studied by transseptal left heart catheterization. *Circulation* 1961;24:267-269.

6. Mitchell JH, Gilmore JP, Sarnoff SJ. The transport function of the atrium: Factors influencing the relation between mean left atrial pressure and left ventricular end-diastolic pressure. *Am J Card* 1962;9:237-247.

7. Crexells C, Chatterjee K, Forrester JS, Dikshit K, Swan HJC. Optimal level of filling pressure in the left side of the heart in acute myocardial infarction. *N Engl J Med* 1973;289:1263-1266.

8. Forrester JS, Diamond G, Chatterjee K, Swan HJC. Medical therapy of acute myocardial infarction by application of hemodynamic subsets. *N Engl J Med* 1976;295:1356-1362 and 1404-1414.

9. Forrester JS, Diamond GA, Swan HJC. Correlative classification of clinical and hemodynamic function after acute myocardial infarction. *Am J Cardiol* 1977;39:137-145.

10. Ganz W, Shah PK, Forrester JS. The role of hemodynamic assessment. In: Fuster V, Ross FL, Topol EJ, eds. Atherosclerosis and Coronary Artery Disease. Philadelphia: Lippincott-Raven, 1996;895-898.

11. McHugh TJ, Adler L, Zion D, Swan HJC, Forrester JS. Simultaneous hemodynamic, radiologic, and physiologic evaluation of left ventricle failure in acute myocardial infarction. *Chest* 1970;58:285-289.

12. McHugh TJ, Forrester JS, Adler L, Zion D, Swan HJC. Pulmonary vascular congestion in acute myocardial infarction: hemodynamic and radiologic correlations. *Ann Intern Med* 1972;76:29-33.

13. Ramo BW, Myers N, Wallace AG, Starmer F, Clark DO, Whalen RE. Hemodynamic findings in 123 patients with acute myocardial infarction on admission. *Circulation* 1970;42:567-577.

14. Chadda KD, Lichstein E, Gupta PK, Choy R. Bradycardia hypotension syndrome in acute myocardial infarction. Reappraisal of the overdrive effects of atropine. *Am J Med* 1975;59:158-164.

15. Robertson D, Hollister AS, Forman MB, Robertson RM. Reflexes unique to myocardial ischemia and infarction. *J Am Coll Cardiol* 1985;5:998.

16. Wei JW, Markis JE, Malagold M, Braunwald E. Cardiovascular reflexes stimulated by reperfusion of ischemic myocardium in acute myocardial infarction. *Circulation* 1983;67:796-801.

17. Come PC, Pitt B. Nitroglycerin induced severe hypotension and bradycardia in patients with acute myocardial infarction. *Circulation* 1976;54:624-628.

18. Gunnar RM. Cardiogenic shock complicating acute myocardial infarction. *Circulation* 1988;78:1508-1510.

19. Eckman MH, Wong JB, Salem DN, Parker SG. Direct angioplasty for acute myocardial infarction: A review of outcomes in clinical subsets. *Ann Intern Med* 1992;117:667-676.

20. Killip T, Kimball JT. Treatment of myocardial infarction in a coronary care unit: A two year experience with 250 patients. *Am J Cardiol* 1967;20:457-464.

21. Gruppo Italiano per lo Studio Streptochinasi Nell'Infarto miocardico (GISSI). Effectiveness of intravenous thrombolytic treatment in acute myocardial infarction. *Lancet* 1986;1:397-402.

22. Alonso DR, Scheidt S, Post M, Killip T. Pathophysiology of cardiogenic shock: quantification of myocardial necrosis, clinical, pathologic, and electrocardiographic correlations. *Circulation* 1973;48:588-596.

23. Lee L, Bates E, Pitt BD, Walton JA, Laufer N, O'Neill WW. Percutaneous transluminal coronary angioplasty improves survival in acute myocardial infarction complicated by cardiogenic shock. *Circulation* 1988;78:1345-1351.

24. Hibbard MD, Holmes DR, Bailey FR, Reeder GS, Bresnalan JF, Gersh BJ. Percutaneous transluminal coronary angioplasty in patients with cardiogenic shock. *J Am Coll Cardiol* 1992;19:639-646.

25. Gacioch GM, Ellis SG, Lee L, Bates ER, Kirsh N, Walton JA, Topol EJ. Cardiogenic shock complicating acute myocardial infarction: The use of coronary angioplasty and the integration of the new support devices into patient management. *J Am Coll Cardiol* 1992;19:647-53.

26. Scheidt S, Ascheim R, Killip T. Shock after acute myocardial infarction: A clinical and hemodynamic profile. *Am J Cardiol* 1970;26:556-564.

27. Gunnar RM, Loeb HS, Pietra RJ, Tobin JR. Hemodynamic measurements in a coronary care unit. *Prog Cardiovasc Dis* 1968;11:29-44.

28. Scheidt S, Wilner G, Mueller H, Summers D, Lesch M, Wolff G, Krakauer J, Rubenfire M, Fleming P, Noon G, Oldham N, Killip T, Kantrowitz A. Intraaortic balloon counter pulsation in cardiogenic shock: Report of a cooperative clinical trial. *N Engl J Med* 1973;288:979-984.

29. Kern MJ, Aguirre FV, Donohue T, Bach R. Coronary hemodynamics. III: Coronary hyperemia. In: Kern MJ, editor. *Hemodynamic Rounds*. New York: Wiley-LISS, Inc., 1993;131-138.

30. Coma-Canella I, Lopez-Sendon J, Nu-nez GL. Subacute left ventricular free wall rupture following acute myocardial infarction: bedside hemodynamics, differential diagnosis, and treatment. *Am Heart J* 1983;106:278-284.

31. Radford MJ, Johnson RA, Daggett WM, et al. Ventricular septal rupture: review of clinical and physiologic features and an analysis of survival. *Circulation* 1981;64:545-553.

32. Grossman W. *Cardiac Catheterization and Angiography*, 2nd ed. Philadelphia: Lea & Febiger, 1980;132-134.

33. Labovitz AJ, Miller LW, Kennedy HL. Mechanical complications of acute myocardial infarction. *Cardiovasc. Rev Rep* 1984;5:948-962.

34. Campion BC, Harrison CE, Giuliani ER, Schattenberg TT, Ellis FH. Ventricular septal defect after myocardial infarction. *Ann Intern Med* 1969;70:251-261.

35. Fuchs RM, Heuser RR, Yin FCP, Brinker JA. Limitations of pulmonary wedge V waves in diagnosing mitral regurgitation. *Am J Cardiol* 1982;49:849-854.

36. Bethen CF, Peter RH, Behar VS, Margolis JR, Kissle JA, Kong Y. The hemodynamic simulation of mitral regurgitation in ventricular septal defect after myocardial infarction. *Cathet Cardiovasc Diagn* 1976;2:97-104.

RIGHT VENTRICULAR INFARCTION
WITH INFERIOR LEFT VENTRICULAR INFARCTION

The hemodynamic features of right ventricular infarction were first described in 1974 by Cohn.[1] Acute right ventricular infarction is usually caused by a proximal occlusion of the right coronary artery.[2] Right ventricular infarction is almost always complicated by inferior left ventricular infarction since the right coronary artery usually also supplies the inferior (diaphragmatic) wall of the left ventricle.[3] Right precordial electrocardiography (leads V_3R to V_6R) can be used to confirm the diagnosis of right ventricular infarction. Lead V_4R is especially useful[4] *(Figure 8.1)*. The hemodynamic profile observed reflects a combination of right ventricular free wall infarction and left ventricular inferior wall infarction.

Physiology of Right Ventricular Infarction

The hemodynamic findings of right ventricular infarction are governed by the infarct size, the degree of right ventricular dilatation, the function of the ventricular septum, the contractile state of the right atrium and the cardiac rhythm.[5] The right ventricle is a thin walled structure with a muscle mass of only one

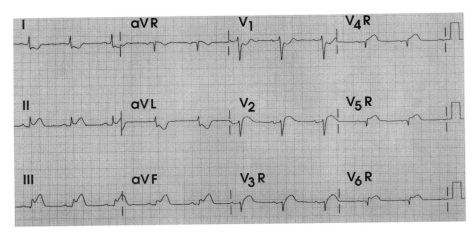

Figure 8.1 Twelve lead electrocardiogram from a patient with an acute inferior myocardial infarction. ST segment elevation is present in the inferior limb leads 2, 3, and aVF. The precordial leads are right sided. Significant ST segment elevation in precordial leads V_3R - V_6R is diagnostic of coincident right ventricular infarction.

sixth that of the left ventricle.[6] Consequently, right ventricular infarction leads to acute right ventricular dilatation. The degree of dilation is limited by the unyielding nature of the normal pericardium resulting in a form of acute pericardial constriction.

The right ventricle shares the interventricular septum with the left ventricle. With right ventricular free wall infarction, the interventricular septum can lend contractile support to the right ventricle, thus limiting the hemodynamic consequences of the infarction.[7] When the infarction also involves the ventricular septum, the consequences are more serious.[8,9] The right coronary artery provides blood supply to a variable portion of the ventricular septum through the posterior descending coronary artery.[10] Therefore, occlusion of the right coronary artery can lead to coincident right ventricular and septal infarction.[5]

The right atrial contractile function and the cardiac rhythm are also important variables. A forceful right atrial contraction can contribute to pulmonary blood flow in these patients.[11]

Unfortunately, right atrial contractile function may be decreased because of coexisting right atrial infarction. It is evident that arrhythmias such as atrial fibrillation and complete heart block are often poorly tolerated because of the loss of right atrial contractile support.[5]

An Overview of Hemodynamic Findings

The right atrial pressure is increased due to right ventricular diastolic dysfunction (decreased compliance). There is a disproportionate increase in the right atrial pressure relative to the wedge pressure.[12] The right atrial pressure waveform resembles that seen with pericardial constriction due to acute right ventricular dilatation.[13,14] The cardiac output and arterial blood pressure may be reduced especially with extensive right ventricular necrosis and interventricular septal necrosis.

Right Atrial Pressure

Typically, the right atrial pressure is elevated to 10 mmHg or greater.[12] The X and Y descents are prominent *(Figure 8.2, Panel A).* This pattern is also seen with pericardial constriction and restrictive cardiomyopathy.[14-16] The prominent X and Y descents cause the right atrial pressure waveform to resemble the letter W or M *(Figure 8.2, Panel A).* Either the X descent or the Y descent may be the dominant negative wave observed during right ventricular infarction and occasionally the two descents are equal.[12,15] Inspiration and volume loading will exaggerate the X and Y descents[17] *(Figure 8.2).* Coma-Canella *et. al.* believe that a dominant Y descent is a marker for a severely injured and noncompliant right ventricle.[15] However, Goldstein and his colleagues have disputed this finding.[18]

It is common to observe an inspiratory increase in the right atrial pressure (Kussmaul's sign, *Figure 8.2, Panel B).* This likely occurs because the injured right heart no longer readily accepts the increased venous return which occurs during spontaneous

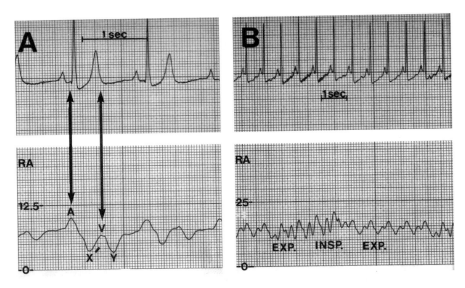

Figure 8.2 (Panels A & B) Right atrial pressure waveform from a patient with right ventricular infarction. **Panel A:** The mean right atrial pressure is elevated at 9 mmHg. The X (**X**) and Y (**Y**) descents are prominent causing the waveform to resemble the letter W. The A wave (**A**) is prominent likely representing augmented right atrial systole. The C wave is trivial. Note the inspiratory exaggeration of the A wave and the X and Y descents present on the first cardiac cycle of this figure. Scale = 0-12.5 mmHg; Paper speed = 25 mm/sec. **Panel B:** Right atrial pressure waveform from a patient with right ventricular infarction. An inspiratory increase in the mean right atrial pressure (Kussmaul's sign) is present. Scale = 0-25 mmHg; Paper speed = 10 mm/sec.

inspiration. Kussmaul's sign can also be observed by carefully examining the neck veins of these patients.[19] The hepatojugular reflux test is often positive in patients with right ventricular infarction *(Figure 8.3)*. The triad of elevated right atrial pressure, prominent X and Y descents, and Kussmaul's sign is also observed with pericardial constriction. As mentioned earlier, right ventricular infarction can be considered a form of pericardial constriction. Right ventricular free wall infarction causes acute right ventricular dilation and the right heart is "constricted" by a normal, but unyielding pericardium.[13,14]

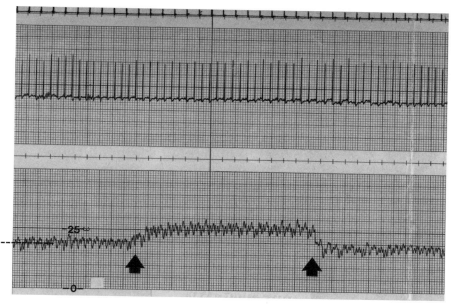

Figure 8.3 Right atrial pressure waveform from a patient with right ventricular infarction. The mean right atrial pressure is elevated at 18 mmHg and a positive hepatojugular reflux test is shown. Manual compression of the abdomen (**first arrow**) causes a persistent elevation of the mean right atrial pressure which resolves upon release (**second arrow**). Scale = 0-25 mmHg; Paper speed = 5 mm/sec.

Right atrial systolic dysfunction may complicate right ventricular infarction, especially when the coronary artery occlusion is proximal and compromises right atrial blood supply.[18] Severe hemodynamic compromise can occur due to the decreased force of right atrial systole.[18] The magnitude of the right atrial A wave (relative to the mean right atrial pressure) provides some information about the atrial contractile function. Patients with small amplitude A waves tend to fare worse than those with augmented A waves[18] *(Figure 8.4)*. Heart block is yet another cause of hemodynamic deterioration during right ventricular infarction. The worsening in hemodynamic status is due primarily to the loss of AV synchrony (not bradycardia) further emphasizing the importance of effective right atrial

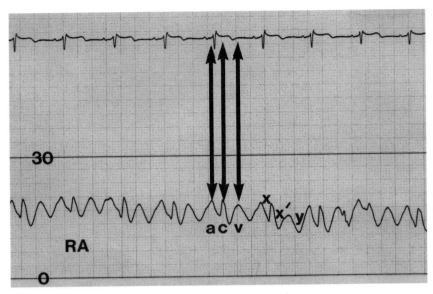

Figure 8.4 Right atrial pressure waveform from a patient with severe right ventricular infarction. The mean right atrial pressure is elevated at 15 mmHg. The A wave (**a**) is attenuated possibly due to right atrial ischemia. The X' (**x'**) and Y (**y**) descents are prominent and vary with respiration. Scale = 0-30 mmHg; Paper speed = 25 mm/sec.

systole.[20] Tricuspid regurgitation can also occur with right ventricular infarction and will alter the right atrial pressure waveform and further raise the right atrial pressure[21] *(Chapter 6).*

Wedge Pressure

The pulmonary capillary wedge pressure is usually elevated because of concomitant inferior-septal left ventricular infarction *(Figure 8.5, Panel A).* Nonetheless, the increase in the right atrial pressure is usually disproportionately greater than the increase in the wedge pressure. The ratio of right atrial pressure/wedge pressure (normal ≤ 0.5) often exceeds 0.75 and may even exceed 1.0 during right ventricular infarction[5,12,14-16] *(Figure 8.5, Panels A & B).* The increase in right atrial pressure relative to left atrial (wedge) pressure can promote right to left shunting across a patent foramen ovale.[22] Serious arterial desaturation can occur.[22]

Pulmonary Artery Pressure and Cardiac Output

Under experimental conditions, the cardiac output and pulmonary artery pressure can be maintained even after destruction of the entire right ventricular free wall.[23,24] In contrast, human right ventricular infarction can be catastrophic.[5,8,9,18] As noted earlier, the explanation for this discrepancy is probably due to the coexistence of septal and left ventricular free wall infarction in human right ventricular infarction. The pulmonary artery pressure is altered by right ventricular infarction. The pulmonary artery diastolic pressure is commonly elevated and parallels the increased wedge pressure caused by inferior wall left ventricular infarction. The right ventricular stroke volume is often reduced causing a decrease in the pulmonary artery pulse pressure[26] *(Figure 8.6)*. With severe right ventricular infarction, the pulmonary artery pulse pressure is so narrowed that it resembles a venous waveform *(Figure 8.6)*. This can make bedside catheter placement difficult. Changing the pressure scale to expand the waveform is helpful *(Figure 8.7, Panels A & B)*. Insertion under fluoroscopy is occasionally necessary. Cardiogenic shock is a common cause of death in these patients.[27]

It is a widely held misconception that volume loading is always beneficial for patients with right ventricular infarction and hemodynamic compromise. In fact, volume loading does not uniformly produce an increase in the cardiac output in these patients.[25] While volume loading can certainly lead to an increase in both the right atrial pressure and the wedge pressure, this may not translate into an improved stroke volume.[25] The increase in the wedge pressure is not associated with an increase in left ventricular volume because of geometric changes in the left ventricle. In fact, volume loading may be harmful if it results in severe peripheral or pulmonary edema. Therefore, it is important to quantitate the effect of volume loading on the stroke volume and cardiac output in these patients.

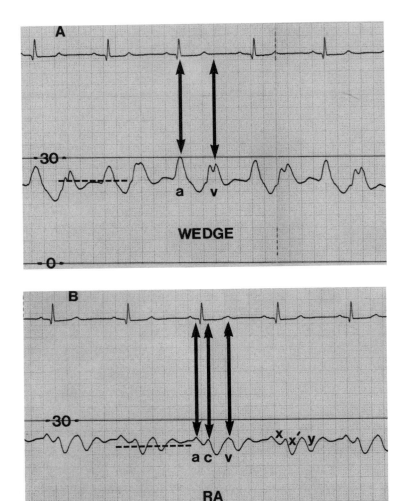

Figure 8.5 (Panels A & B): Wedge pressure and right atrial pressure waveforms from a patient with right ventricular infarction.

Panel A: The mean wedge pressure is elevated at 23 mmHg due to inferior left ventricular infarction.

Panel B: The mean right atrial pressure is elevated at 23 mmHg. The ratio of right atrial to wedge pressure is 1.0. Prominent X'(**x'**) and Y (**y**) descents are present. An H wave is visible following the Y descent because of sinus bradycardia. Scale = 0-30 mmHg; Paper speed = 25 mm/sec.

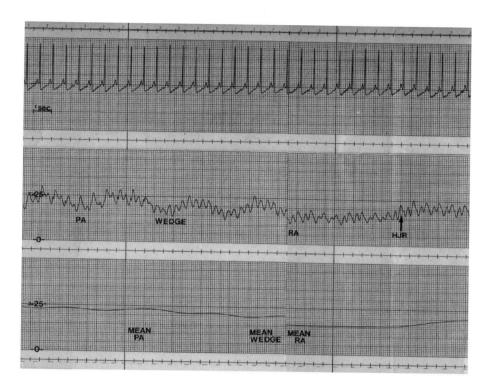

Figure 8.6 Pulmonary artery (**PA**), wedge, and right atrial (**RA**) pressure recordings from a patient with severe right ventricular infarction. The pulmonary artery pulse pressure is narrow because of reduced right ventricular stroke volume and the waveform resembles that of a venous tracing. The mean wedge pressure is elevated at 20 mmHg because of inferior wall left ventricular infarction. The mean right atrial pressure is elevated at 16 mmHg and the ratio of right atrial to wedge pressure is 0.8. The mean pressures in the pulmonary artery, wedge, and right atrium are therefore quite similar. In this situation, catheter placement can be very difficult without fluoroscopy. Scale = 0-25 mmHg; Paper speed = 5 mm/sec.

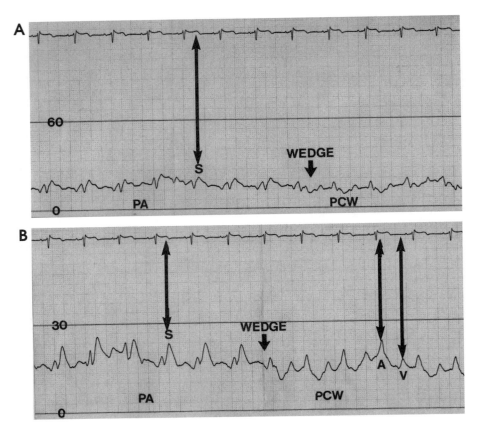

Figure 8.7 (Panels A & B): Pulmonary artery and wedge pressure waveforms from a patient with right ventricular infarction recorded on different pressure scales.

Panel A : The pressure scale is 0-60 mmHg. The pulmonary artery pulse pressure is reduced because of decreased right ventricular stroke volume. It is difficult to appreciate the change from pulmonary artery (**PA**) to wedge (**PCW**) in this tracing. S = pulmonary artery systolic wave; Arrow = balloon inflation; Paper speed = 25 mm/sec.

Panel B : The pressure scale is now 0-30 mmHg. The pulmonary artery (**PA**) pressure waveform and transition to wedge (**PCW**) waveform are much easier to recognize. The A and V waves can now be identified in the wedge waveform. S = Pulmonary artery systolic wave; Arrow = balloon inflation; Paper speed = 25 mm/sec.

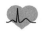 **Key Points: Right Ventricular Infarction**

- The right atrial pressure is elevated to ≥ 10 mmHg. The right atrial pressure waveform resembles pericardial constriction with prominent x and y descents. Kussmaul's sign is common and the hepatojugular reflux test is positive.

- The right atrial pressure is elevated out of proportion to the wedge pressure. The ratio of right atrial pressure/wedge pressure exceeds 0.75.

- The pulmonary artery pulse pressure is decreased due to decreased right ventricular stroke volume.

- Septal infarction, right atrial infarction, heart block, atrial fibrillation, and tricuspid regurgitation are variables which can cause hemodynamic deterioration in these patients.

- Paradoxical embolization and right to left shunting can occur if the right atrial pressure exceeds the wedge pressure.

Chapter 8 References

1. Cohn JN, Guiha NH, Broder MI, Limas CJ. Right ventricular infarction: Clinical and hemodynamic features. *Am J Cardiol* 1974;33:209-214.

2. Haupt HM, Hutchins GM, Moore GW. Right ventricular infarction: role of the moderator band artery in determining infarct size. *Circulation* 1983;67:1268-72.

3. Isner JM, Roberts WC. Right ventricular infarction complicating left ventricular infarction secondary to coronary heart disease: frequency, location, associated findings, and significance from analysis of 236 necropsy patients with acute or healed myocardial infarction. *Am J Cardiol* 1978; 42:885-94.

4. Klein HO, Tordjman T, Ninio R, Sareli P, Oren V, Lang R, Gefen J, Pauzner C, Di Segni E, David D, Kaplinsky E. The early recognition of right ventricular infarction: Diagnostic accuracy of the electrocardiographic V_4R lead. *Circulation* 1983;67:558-65.

5. Kinch PA, Ryan TJ. Right ventricular infarction. *N Engl J Med* 1994;330-1211-1217.

6. Dell'Italia LJ. The right ventricle: anatomy, physiology, and clinical importance. *Curr Prob Cardiol* 1991;16:657-720.

7. Sharkey SW, Shelley W, Carlyle PF, Rysavy J, Cohn JN. M-mode and two-dimensional echocardiographic analysis of the septum in experimental right ventricular infarction: Correlation with hemodynamic alterations. *Am Heart J* 1985;110:1210-1218.

8. Goldstein JA, Harada A, Yagi Y, Barzilai B, Cox JL. Hemodynamic importance of systolic ventricular interaction, augmented right atrial contractility, and atrioventricular synchrony in acute right ventricular dysfunction. *J Am Coll Cardiol* 1990;16:181-189.

9. Mikell F, Asinger R, Hodges M. Functional consequences of interventricular septal involvement in right ventricular infarction: Echocardiographic, clinical, and hemodynamic observations. *Am Heart J* 1983;105:393-401.

10. Farrer-Brown G. Vascular pattern of myocardium of right ventricle of human heart. *Br Heart J* 1965;30:679-686.

11. Lopez-Sendon J, Garcia AG, Marti JS, Roldan I. Complete pulmonic valve opening during atrial contraction after right ventricular infarction. *Am J Cardiol* 1985;56:486-487.

12. Lopez-Sendon J, Coma-Canella I, Gamallo C. Sensitivity and specificity of hemodynamic criteria in the diagnosis of acute right ventricular infarction. *Circulation* 1981;64:515-525.

13. Shabetai R. The pericardium: An essay on some recent developments. *Am J Cardiol* 1978;42:1036-43.

14. Lorell B, Leimbach RC, Pohost AM, Gold HK, Dinsmore RE, Hutter AM, Pastore JO, DeSanctis RW. Right ventricular infarction: Clinical diagnosis and differentiation from cardiac tamponade and pericardial constriction. *Am J Cardiol* 1979;43:465-471.

15. Coma-Canella I, Lopez-Sendon J. Ventricular compliance in ischemic right ventricular dysfunction. *Am J Cardiol* 1980;45:555-61.

16. Lloyd EA, Gersh BJ, Kenelly BM. Hemodynamic spectrum of "dominant"

right ventricular infarction in 19 patients. *Am J Cardiol* 1981;48:1016-1022.

17. Dell'Italia LJ, Starling MR, Crawford MH, Boros BL, Claudhuri TK, O'Rourke RA, Heyl B, Amon W. Right ventricular infarction: Identification by hemodynamic measurements before and after volume loading and correlation with noninvasive techniques. *J Am Coll Cardiol* 1984;4:931-939.

18. Goldstein JA, Barzilai B, Rosamond TL, Eisenberg PR, Jaffe AS. Determinants of hemodynamic compromise with severe right ventricular infarction. *Circulation* 1990;82:359-368.

19. Dell'Italia LJ, Starling MR, O'Rourke RA. Physical examination for exclusion of hemodynamically important right ventricular infarction. *Ann Intern Med* 1983;99:608-611.

20. Topol ES, Goldschlager N, Ports TA, DiCarlo LA, Schiller NB, Botvinick EH, Chatterjee K. Hemodynamic benefit of atrial pacing in right ventricular myocardial infarction. *Ann Intern Med* 1982;96:594-97.

21. MacAllister RG, Friesinger GC, Sinclair-Smith BC. Tricuspid regurgitation following inferior myocardial infarction. *Arch Intern Med* 1976;136:95-99.

22. Manno BV, Bemis CE, Carver J, Mintz GS. Right ventricular infarction complicated by right to left shunt. *J Am Coll Cardiol* 1983;1:554-557.

23. Starr J, Jeffers WA, Meade RN. The absence of conspicuous increments of venous pressure after severe damage to the right ventricle of the dog with a discussion of the relation between clinical congestive failure and heart disease. *Am Heart J* 1943;26:291-301.

24. Guiha NH, Limas CJ, Cohn JN. Predominant right ventricular dysfunction after right ventricular destruction in the dog. *Am J Cardiol* 1974;33:254-258.

25. Dell'Italia LJ, Starling MR, Blumhardt R, Lasher JC, O'Rourke RA. Comparative effects of volume loading, dobutamine and nitroprusside in patients with predominant right ventricular infarction. *Circulation* 1985;72:1327-1335.

26. Coma-Canella I, Lopez-Sendon J, Gamallo C. Low output syndrome in right ventricular infarction. *Am Heart J* 1979;98:613-620.

27. Zehender M, Kasper W, Kauder E, Schönthaler M, Geibel A, Olschewski M, Just H. Right ventricular infarction as an independent predictor of prognosis after acute inferior myocardial infarction. *N Engl J Med* 1992;328:981-8.

ACUTE LEFT VENTRICULAR ISCHEMIA

M yocardial ischemia can complicate many serious illnesses since coronary artery disease is so common in the intensive care unit population. It can be difficult to recognize the presence of myocardial ischemia; it is often painless and short lived. In the intensive care unit, intermittent left ventricular ischemia may manifest itself clinically as congestive heart failure. Recurrent painless ischemia is one of the causes of refractory respiratory failure.[1] Myocardial ischemia is evanescent and continuous recording of hemodynamic parameters is necessary to detect its presence.

Hemodynamic Consequences of Acute Ischemia

Acute left ventricular ischemia causes immediate impairment of both systolic and diastolic myocardial function.[2] The hemodynamic changes occur in both painful and painless ischemia.[3-5] The diastolic dysfunction leads to an increase in the left ventricular end diastolic pressure[3-7] *(Figure 9.1)*. The increase in the left ventricular end diastolic pressure is transmitted to the left atrium causing an increase in the wedge pressure.[7] Eventually, the elevated left ventricular filling pressure leads to pulmonary

Baseline   **Ischemia**

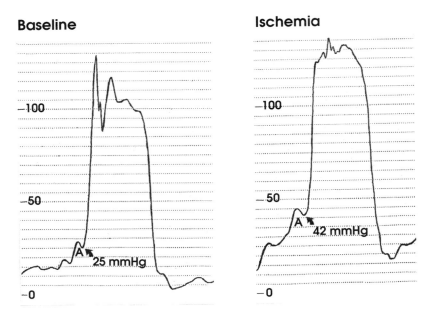

Figure 9.1 Left ventricular pressure recording at baseline (**left**) and during spontaneous myocardial ischemia (**right**). At baseline, the left ventricular end diastolic pressure is 25 mmHg (**arrow**). A modest A wave (**A**) is present on the pressure tracing. During ischemia, the left ventricular diastolic pressure increases significantly. The left ventricular end diastolic pressure (**arrow**) is now 42 mmHg due in part to an exaggeration of the A wave. Note also that the left ventricular systolic pressure increases during ischemia in this patient who is experiencing significant chest pain.
Scale = 0-100 mmHg; Paper speed = 50 mm/sec.

venous congestion.[1-3] When myocardial ischemia causes an elevation of the wedge pressure to ≥ 25 mmHg, overt pulmonary edema occurs.[8,9] The rate of formation of interstitial and alveolar pulmonary edema may be very rapid during periods of elevated pulmonary capillary wedge pressure.[10] In contrast, removal rate of the edema fluid is often relatively slow once the elevated wedge pressure has returned to normal.[11] As a result, the clinical and radiographic effects of the pulmonary edema may linger long after hemodynamic measurements have returned to normal.

Baseline

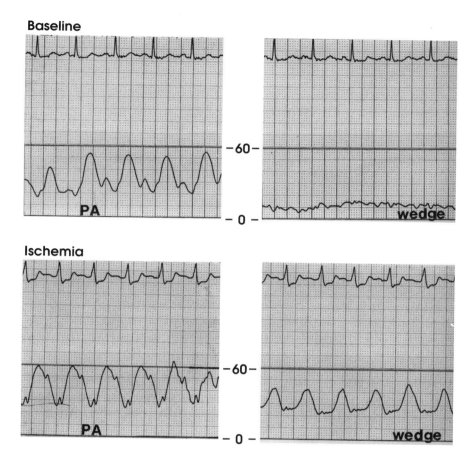

Figure 9.2 Recording of pulmonary artery pressure (**PA**), wedge pressure (**wedge**) and Lead II electrocardiogram at baseline (**top**) and during ischemia (**bottom**). At baseline, the heart rate is 96 beats/min, and the Lead II ST-segment is isoelectric. The pulmonary artery pressure is 50/20 mmHg and the mean wedge pressure is 15 mmHg. During spontaneous ischemia, the heart rate is 110 beats/min and there is 2 mm (0.2 mV) ST-segment depression in Lead II. The pulmonary artery pressure is 62/26 mmHg and the mean wedge pressure is 34 mmHg. During ischemia, the pulmonary artery diastolic pressure significantly underestimates the mean wedge pressure because of the presence of a large V wave. Scale = 0-60 mmHg.

The pulmonary artery pressure increases during acute ischemia because of the sudden increase in the left ventricular end diastolic pressure and the wedge pressure *(Figure 9.2)*. Baseline measurements of the pulmonary artery pressure and the wedge pressure are deceiving and may be normal *(Table 9.1)*. During acute ischemia striking increases in the heart rate, pulmonary artery pressure and wedge pressure may occur *(Table 9.1)*. Continuous recording of the pulmonary artery pressure can be used to detect ischemic mediated increases in the left ventricular end diastolic pressure[12-16] *(Figure 9.3)*. At the same time, measurement of the pulmonary artery diastolic pressure provides an assessment of the physiologic consequences of such episodes with respect to pulmonary congestion. Transient pulmonary artery hypertension can occur with stresses other than ischemia. It is therefore necessary to continuously record the ST-segment of the electrocardiogram to prove that myocardial ischemia is the cause of observed increases in the pulmonary artery pressure[1] *(Figure 9.4)*.

Table 9.1 Hemodynamic Parameters at Baseline & During Ischemia*		
	Baseline	**Ischemia**
HR (beats/min)	77 (55-90)	95 (67-114)
PAP systolic (mmHg)	34 (27-42)	72 (56-80)
PAP diastolic (mmHg)	19 (16-24)	41 (38-45)
PCW (mmHg)	14 (11-17)	40 (31-48)

*The above data was collected from patients presenting with ischemia mediated acute pulmonary edema.

Data presented are mean and (range). HR = heart rate; PAP = pulmonary artery pressure; PCW = pulmonary capillary wedge pressure.

Figure 9.3 Continuous recording of heart rate and pulmonary artery pressures from a patient with recurrent acute pulmonary edema.
Top: Before angioplasty (PTCA), multiple episodes of painless pulmonary artery hypertension and sinus tachycardia are present. Each episode was associated with ST-segment depression in leads V_1 - V_6.

Before PTCA

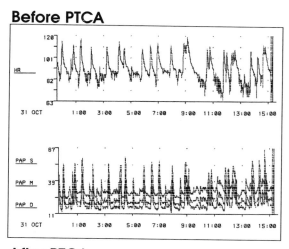

Bottom: After PTCA, the episodic pulmonary hypertension is gone. The pulmonary edema resolved and the patient was extubated. HR = heart rate (scale is in beats/min); PAP = pulmonary artery pressure; S = systolic; M = mean; D = diastolic (scale is in mmHg). Time displayed is military time. (From Sharkey SW, Aberg NB, *Am Heart J* 1995; 129:189, with permission).

After PTCA

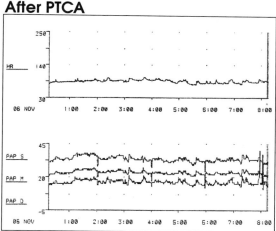

Wedge Pressure and Pulmonary Artery Pressure

During acute ischemia, both the A and V waves of the wedge pressure waveform are accentuated because the increased left atrial pressure distends the pulmonary venous channels allowing more effective transmission of all left atrial mechanical events. Even in the absence of significant mitral regurgitation, the V wave of the wedge pressure is often increased relative to the A wave because of ischemia mediated noncompliance of the left heart.

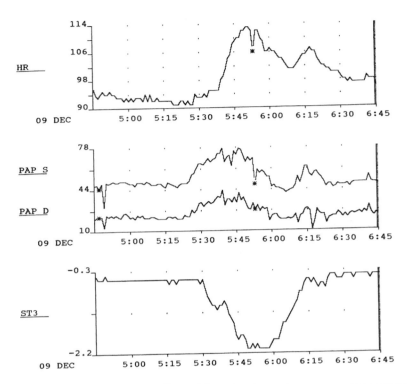

Figure 9.4 Continuous recording of heart rate, pulmonary artery pressure, and ST-segment deviation in lead V$_3$ over 2 hours. An episode of spontaneous ischemia occurs at about 05:30. At baseline (05:15), the heart rate is 94 beats/min, the pulmonary artery pressure is 46/21 mmHg, and ST-segment depression of 0.5 mm (0.05 mV) is present. During peak ischemia, the heart rate is 112 beats/min, the pulmonary artery pressure is 78/44 mmHg and ST-segment depression of 2.1 mm (0.21 mV) is present. Careful inspection of this recording reveals that the change in the pulmonary artery pressure and the ST-segment precede the increase in the heart rate. HR = heart rate (scale is 90 to 114 beats/min); PAP = pulmonary artery pressure; S = systolic and D = diastolic (scale is 10 to 78 mmHg); ST3 = ST-segment in Lead V$_3$ (scale is -0.3 to -2.2 mm, 1 mm = 0.1 mV).

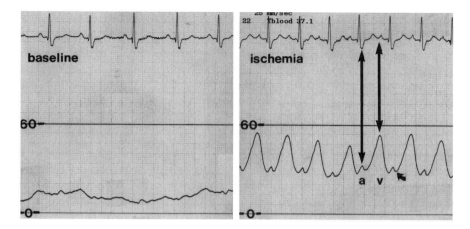

Figure 9.5 Wedge pressure waveform at baseline (**left**) and during spontaneous myocardial ischemia (**right**). The patient was intubated because of severe pulmonary edema. The episodes of ischemia were painless. At baseline, the mean wedge pressure is 14 mmHg. The A and V waves are not obvious. During ischemia, the mean wedge pressure is 48 mmHg with large V waves suggesting the presence of concomitant acute mitral regurgitation. Note also that both the A (**a**) and V (**v**) waves are transmitted to the wedge pressure waveform with greater fidelity because the increased left atrial pressure has "opened" more pulmonary venous channels. The mean wedge pressure will likely overestimate the left ventricular end diastolic pressure due to the large V wave (*see also Chapter 5*). The post A wave wedge pressure (curved **arrow**) is 29 mmHg and provides a better estimate of the actual left ventricular end diastolic pressure in this patient. However, the mean wedge pressure is still the more clinically relevant parameter in this patient with severe pulmonary edema. Scale = 0-60 mmHg; Paper speed = 25 mm/sec.

The magnitude of the increase in the wedge pressure depends on the duration of the ischemia, the baseline left ventricular function, and the amount of myocardium involved. Papillary muscle ischemia can cause a profound increase in the mean wedge pressure because of transient severe mitral regurgitation.[17] In this setting, it is common to observe a mean wedge pressure exceeding 30 mmHg together with a giant V wave (*Figure 9.5*).

The increase in the wedge pressure is transmitted to the pulmonary circulation causing an increase in the pulmonary artery systolic and diastolic pressures.[18,19] During ischemia, the pulmonary artery diastolic pressure may significantly under-estimate the mean wedge pressure if a large V wave is present in the wedge waveform (*Figure 9.2*). It is quite common to observe an increase in the heart rate of 10-15 beats/min in response to an episode of ischemia even in the absence of symptoms[5,18,20] (*Figure 9.4*). In general, painful ischemia produces a greater hemodynamic derangement than does painless ischemia.[5]

The right atrial pressure is not sensitive to episodes of left ventricular ischemia. However, the right atrial pressure waveform may be altered if right ventricular ischemia also occurs (*Chapter 8*). The right atrial waveform will also change if sinus tachycardia or other arrhythmias complicate the ischemic episode. The aortic pressure is insensitive to myocardial ischemia and may either decrease or increase.[5,7,18-20] In the hospitalized patient, an increase in the arterial pressure is usually not the trigger for ischemic episodes.[20]

Clinical Observations

Most episodes of myocardial ischemia will not cause clinically important hemodynamic changes. In an occasional patient, recurrent ischemia causes profound heart failure (especially acute pulmonary edema). These patients are often elderly and present with acute dyspnea and pulmonary edema requiring mechanical ventilation.[1] Anginal pain is uncommon or absent. These patients often have evidence of previous myocardial infarction by history or electrocardiogram. Left ventricular dysfunction with one or more wall motion abnormalities and mild to moderate mitral regurgitation is usually present on a baseline two-dimensional echocardiogram. Continuous hemodynamic monitoring typically reveals multiple episodes of profound pulmonary hypertension and ST-segment deviation (*Figure.9.3*). This behavior is reminiscent of the cyclic decreases in coronary artery blood flow which can be observed experimentally in the presence of a critical coronary stenosis.[21] Patients with ischemia mediated acute heart failure typically have extensive 3-vessel coronary artery disease.[22-26] In addition, these patients often have a unique pattern of 3-vessel coronary artery disease with an occlusion of at least one major vessel, extensive collateral connections, and a severe stenosis in a coronary artery that provides collateral flow to the occluded vessel.[1] This constellation of severe coronary artery disease is more likely to occur in elderly patients. A sudden decrease in blood flow through the stenotic collateral supporting vessel or a sudden increase in myocardial oxygen demand could trigger the profound hemodynamic changes observed in Table 9.1. Revascularization with coronary angioplasty or bypass surgery is often effective therapy[2,7] (*Figure 9.3*).

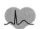 **Key Points: Acute Left Ventricular Ischemia**

- Acute ischemia elevates the left ventricular end diastolic pressure. This in turn leads to an increase in the wedge pressure and the pulmonary artery pressure. Continuous monitoring techniques are necessary to detect these changes.

- Most episodes of acute ischemia do not cause hemodynamic compromise. In an occasional patient, myocardial ischemia can cause profound heart failure (pulmonary edema).

- Papillary muscle ischemia can cause intermittent severe mitral regurgitation. In this setting, the mean wedge pressure commonly exceeds 30 mmHg with a giant V wave present. In the presence of a large V wave, the pulmonary artery diastolic pressure significantly underestimates the mean wedge pressure.

- Transient elevations of the wedge pressure and pulmonary artery pressure can be caused by stresses other than acute ischemia. Continuous recording of the ST-segment together with hemodynamic parameters is a helpful method for proving the presence of intermittent ischemia.

Chapter 9 References

1. Sharkey SW, Aberg NB. Hemodynamic evidence of painless myocardial ischemia with acute pulmonary edema in coronary disease. *Am Heart J* 1995;129:188-91.

2. Hillis LD, Braunwald E. Myocardial ischemia. *N Engl J Med* 1977;296:971-976.

3. Müller O, Rørvik K. Haemodynamic consequences of coronary heart disease with observations during anginal pain and on the effect of nitroglycerine. *Br Heart J* 1958;20:302-310.

4. Figueras J, Singh B, Ganz W, Charuzi Y, Swan H. Mechanism of rest and nocturnal angina: observations during continuous hemodynamic and electrocardiographic monitoring. *Circulation* 1979;59:955-68.

5. Chierchia S, Lazzari M, Freedman B, Brunelli C, Maseri A. Impairment of myocardial perfusion and function during painless myocardial ischemia. *J Am Coll Cardiol* 1983;1:924-930.

6. Grossman W, McLaurin LP. Diastolic properties of the left ventricle. *Ann Inter Med* 1976;84:316-326.

7. Parker JO. Hemodynamic and metabolic changes during myocardial ischemia. *Arch Intern Med* 1972;129:790-798.

8. McHugh TJ, Forrester JS, Adler L, Zion D, Swan HJC. Pulmonary vascular congestion in acute myocardial infarction: hemodynamic and radiologic correlations. *Ann Intern Med* 1972;76:29-33.

9. Guyton A, Lindsey AW. Effect of elevated left atrial pressure and decreased plasma protein concentration on the development of pulmonary edema. *Circ Res* 1959;7:649-57.

10. Minnear FL, Barie PS, Malik AB. Effects of large, transient increases in pulmonary vascular pressures on lung fluid balance. *J Appl Physiol* 1983;55:983.

11. Cross CE, Shaver JA, Wilson RJ, Robin ED. Mitral stenosis and pulmonary fibrosis: Special reference to pulmonary edema and lung lymphatic function. *Arch Intern Med* 1970;125:248.

12. Jenkin BS, Bradley RD, Branthwaite MA. Evaluation of pulmonary arterial end diastolic pressure as an indirect estimate of left atrial mean pressure. *Circulation* 1970;42:75-8.

13. Bouchard RJ, Gault JH, Ross J. Evaluation of pulmonary arterial end diastolic pressure as an estimate of left ventricular end diastolic pressure in patients with normal and abnormal left ventricular performance. *Circulation* 1971;44:1072-9.

14. Forsberg SA. Relations between pressure in pulmonary artery, left atrium, and left ventricle with special reference to events at end diastole. *Brit Heart J* 1971;33:494-9.

15. Levy RD, Shapiro LM, Wright C, Mockus LJ, Fox KM. The hemodynamic significance of asymptomatic ST segment depression assessed by ambulatory pulmonary artery pressure monitoring. *Br Heart J* 1986; 56:526-30.

16. Levy RD, Cunningham D, Shapiro LM, Wright C, Markus L, Fox KM. Continuous ambulatory pulmonary artery pressure monitoring: a new method using a transducer-tipped catheter and a simple recording system. *Brit Heart J* 1986;55:336-43.

17. Brody W, Criley JM. Intermittent severe mitral regurgitation. Hemodynamic studies in a patient with recurrent left-sided heart failure. *N Engl J Med* 1970; 283:673-676.

18. Roughgarden JW. Circulatory changes associated with spontaneous angina pectoris. *Am J Med* 1966;41:947-961.

19. Guazzi M, Polese A, Fiorentini C, Magrini F, Olivari MI, Bartorelli C. Left and right heart haemodynamics during spontaneous angina pectoris: comparison between angina with ST segment depression and angina with ST segment elevation. *Br Heart J* 1975;37:401-413.

20. Chierchia S, Brunelli C, Simonetti I, Lazzari M, Maseri A. Sequence of events in angina at rest: primary reduction in coronary flow. *Circulation* 1980;61:759-768.

21. Folts JD, Crowell EB, Rowe GG. Platelet aggregation in partially obstructed vessels and its elimination with aspirin. *Circulation* 1976;54:365-70.

22. Goldberger JJ, Peled HB, Stroh JA, Cohen MN, Frishman WH. Prognostic factors in acute pulmonary edema. *Arch Intern Med* 1986;146:489.

23. Clark LT, Garfein OB, Dwyer EM. Acute pulmonary edema due to ischemic heart disease without accompanying myocardial infarction. *Am J Med* 1983;75:332-6.

24. Dodek A, Kassebaum DG, Bristow JD. Pulmonary edema in coronary artery disease without cardiomegaly. *N Engl J Med* 1972;286:1347-50.

25. Graham SP, Vetrovec GW. Comparison of angiographic findings and demographic variables in patients with coronary artery disease presenting with acute pulmonary edema versus those presenting with chest pain. *Am J Cardiol* 1991;68:1614-8.

26. Lee FA, Cabin HS, Francis CK. The syndrome of flash pulmonary edema: clinical definition and angiographic findings. *J Am Coll Cardiol* 1988;11:151A.

27. Kunis R, Greenberg H. Yeoh CB, et al. Coronary revascularization for recurrent pulmonary edema in elderly patients with ischemic heart disease and preserved ventricular function. *N Engl J Med* 1985;313:1207-10.

10

CHRONIC CONGESTIVE HEART FAILURE

Congestive heart failure is the unfortunate final outcome for a number of heart diseases. In contrast to patients with acute heart failure, the physical examination and chest x-ray are of limited value in accurately predicting the hemodynamic status of patients with chronic congestive heart failure.[1-3] In one study, physical examination evidence specific for pulmonary congestion was absent in 44% of patients with pulmonary capillary wedge pressures $\geq$ 35 mmHg.[1] Similarly, chest x-ray evidence of an increased wedge pressure (interstitial or alveolar edema) may be masked by the increased lymphatic drainage which occurs in patients with chronic heart failure.[4-6] Hemodynamic monitoring is often necessary to guide therapy in patients admitted to the hospital with refractory heart failure.[7-9] These patients are highly selected and the hemodynamic data observed are not representative of the chronic heart failure population at large. The hemodynamic findings discussed in this chapter pertain to patients with chronic congestive heart failure in the setting of a dilated heart with poor systolic function (i.e., dilated cardiomyopathy).

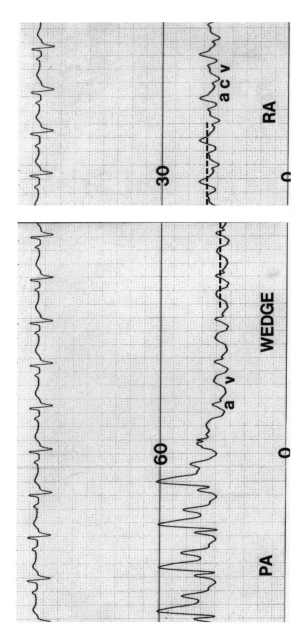

Figure 10.1 Pulmonary artery (**PA**), wedge, and right atrial (**RA**) pressure waveforms from a patient with chronic congestive heart failure. The pulmonary artery pressure is 61/33 mmHg; the mean wedge pressure is 31 mmHg; and the mean right atrial pressure is 19 mmHg (note: the right atrial pressure scale is 0-30 mmHg). The ratio of the mean right atrial pressure/mean wedge pressure is nearly normal (0.6) in this patient without significant tricuspid regurgitation. The pulmonary artery diastolic pressure and the mean wedge pressure are nearly identical. The wedge pressure A (**a**) and V (**v**) waves are of similar amplitude. Mitral regurgitation was absent on echocardiography. Despite a mean wedge pressure of 31 mmHg, the patient was comfortable lying flat in bed. Scale = 0-60 mmHg (PA) and 0-30 mmHg (RA); Paper speed = 25 mm/sec.

Right Atrial Pressure, Wedge Pressure & Pulmonary Artery Pressure
Typically, all intracardiac pressures are elevated to a varying degree
(Figure 10.1). The mean right atrial pressure and the mean wedge
pressure are subject to the influence of any coexisting tricuspid or
mitral regurgitation respectively. Atrial and ventricular arrhythmias
are common in these patients and will alter the right atrial and
wedge pressure waveforms.

The mean right atrial pressure in patients hospitalized with
severe heart failure is 9-12 mmHg (range 2-38 mmHg).[1-3,7-9] The
mean wedge pressure is 21-30 mmHg (range 8-44 mmHg).[1-3,7-9]
The mean pulmonary artery pressure is 33 mmHg.[1-3,7-9]
Typical hemodynamic measurements observed with chronic
congestive heart failure are shown in Figure 10.1. Patients with
chronic heart failure generally have higher intracardiac
pressures than do patients with acute heart failure. In one
study, the mean wedge pressure was ≥ 35 mmHg in 36% of
patients hospitalized with severe chronic congestive failure.[1]
In comparison, the mean wedge pressure of patients with acute
myocardial infarction and cardiogenic shock is typically 18-28
mmHg[10] *(Chapter 7)*.

It is important to note the relation between the mean right
atrial pressure and the mean wedge pressure. In many patients
with chronic heart failure, the usual ratio of right atrial
pressure/wedge pressure of ≤ 0.5 is observed. However, it is not
uncommon to find the ratio to exceed 0.5 because of right
ventricular dilatation and severe tricuspid regurgitation.[11] In
some patients, right heart failure may predominate resulting in a
right atrial pressure greater than the wedge pressure. The right
atrial pressure waveform will have the features typical of
tricuspid regurgitation in this subset of patients *(Figure 10.2 &
Chapter 6)*. It is rare for the mean right atrial pressure to actually
exceed the mean wedge pressure unless a complication such as
pulmonary embolism has occurred *(Chapter 13)*.

The wedge pressure waveform is dominated by the V wave.
The V wave is prominent because of noncompliance of the left

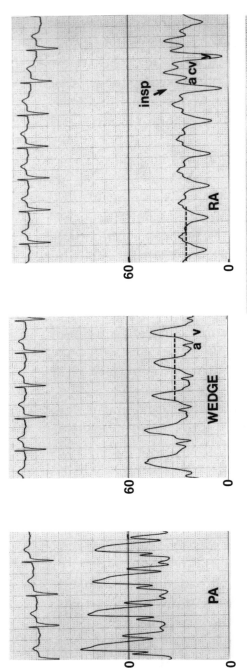

Figure 10.2 Hemodynamic data recorded from a patient with refractory heart failure due to ischemic heart disease and severe mitral regurgitation. Sinus tachycardia 100 beats/min is present. The pulmonary artery (**PA**) pressure is markedly elevated (83/35 mmHg); the mean wedge pressure is 32 mmHg with a V (**v**) wave of 47 mmHg; the mean right atrial (**RA**) pressure is 26 mmHg. The ratio of mean RA pressure/mean wedge pressure is increased (0.7) because of severe tricuspid regurgitation. The right atrial pressure waveform is typical of tricuspid regurgitation with a prominent CV wave and steep Y descent (**y**). Note that inspiration (**insp**) accentuates both the positive waves (A, C, V) and the negative waves (X, X', Y).

The wedge pressure waveform is dominated by the V wave in part because of significant mitral regurgitation. With a large V wave, the pulmonary artery diastolic pressure should be significantly less than the mean wedge pressure (*Chapter 5*). In this patient, the pulmonary artery diastolic pressure exceeds the mean wedge pressure because of increased pulmonary vascular resistance. A lung scan revealed no evidence for pulmonary embolism. Despite a mean wedge pressure of 32 mmHg, the patient was comfortable lying flat in bed. The thermodilution cardiac output (CO) curve is distorted by tricuspid regurgitation. The computer generated cardiac output (3.4 L/min) is probably inaccurate. Scale = 0-60 mmHg; Paper speed = 25 mm/sec.

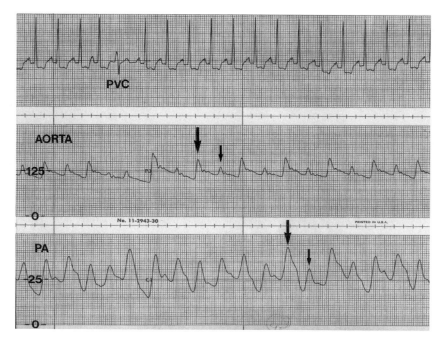

Figure 10.3 Aortic and pulmonary artery (**PA**) pressure waveforms from a patient with severe congestive heart failure. A premature ventricular contraction (**PVC**) initiates pulsus alternans (**arrows**) which is visible in both the aortic and pulmonary artery tracings. Scale = 0-125 mmHg (aorta) and 0-25 mmHg (PA); Paper speed = 25 mm/sec.

heart although it is also common to find some degree of mitral regurgitation in these patients.[12] Moderate pulmonary hypertension is the rule. The close relation between the pulmonary artery diastolic pressure and the mean wedge pressure is maintained *(Figure 10.1)*. If the pulmonary artery diastolic pressure exceeds the mean wedge pressure by ≥ 5 mmHg, the presence of a complication such as pulmonary embolism should be considered *(Chapter 13)*. The pulmonary artery pulse pressure may be narrow in the presence of a low stroke volume.

Aortic Pressure

The aortic pressure may be normal or even high in the face of severe congestive heart failure. A decrease in the aortic pulse

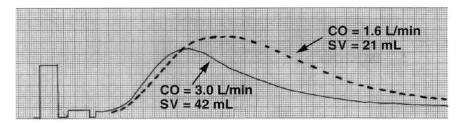

Figure 10.4 Superimposed cardiac output curves before and after therapy for refractory heart failure. At baseline (**dashed line**) the cardiac output is 1.6 L/min due to a profound decrease in the stroke volume (21 mL/beat). After treatment with intravenous inotropic drugs (**solid line**), the cardiac output is now 3.0 L/min. The improved cardiac output is primarily due to doubling of the stroke volume (42 mL/beat). Calibration artifact is -0.5°C.

pressure correlates with a decrease in the cardiac index.[13,14] Occasionally, pulsus alternans occurs in the final stages of congestive heart failure *(Figure 10.3)*.[15]

Cardiac Output/Index

As expected, the cardiac output and index are usually reduced with the average being 3.0 L/min and 1.6 L/min/m² respectively.[8] The low cardiac output is due largely to a significant reduction in the stroke volume. An occasional patient will have a marked reduction in the cardiac index to levels as low as 1.0 to 1.5 L/min/m² *(Figure 10.4)*. In acute heart failure, patients with a cardiac index below 1.8 L/min/m² exhibit clinical cardiogenic shock *(Chapter 7)*.[10] Patients with chronic heart failure adapt to a low cardiac index primarily by increasing the tissue extraction of oxygen from hemoglobin, resulting in a decrease in the mixed venous (pulmonary artery) oxygen saturation.[16]

In patients with severe heart failure, the thermodilution measurement of the cardiac output is susceptible to error. The presence of significant tricuspid regurgitation renders the thermodilution method inaccurate.[17] Significant tricuspid

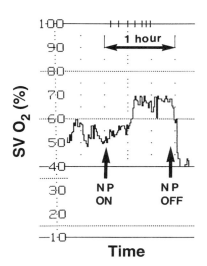

Figure 10.5 Effect of nitroprusside therapy for congestive heart failure on the pulmonary artery oxygen saturation (**SV O$_2$**). Before nitroprusside, the SV O$_2$ is 55%. During nitroprusside infusion (**NP on**), the SV O$_2$ rises abruptly to 70% reflecting an increase in the forward cardiac output. After infusion (**NP off**), the SV O$_2$ drops reflecting a sudden decrease in the cardiac output.

regurgitation can be recognized by the characteristic right atrial pressure waveform and the prolonged decay phase of the thermodilution curve *(Figure 10.2)*. Arrhythmias are another potential source of error. The thermodilution method samples blood flow during only a few heart beats and extrapolates this measurement to a one minute period. If a ventricular or atrial arrhythmia occurs during the injection and sampling period, the cardiac output measurement may not be representative of the patient's steady state cardiac output. Atrial fibrillation is a major offender, especially when the R-R intervals are varying widely. It is therefore important to note the heart rate and rhythm during the injection and sampling phase of the thermodilution measurement. The Fick method provides an alternate means of measuring the cardiac output when either tricuspid regurgitation or an arrhythmia invalidate the thermodilution method *(Chapter 3)*. This method is tedious and therefore impractical for making serial measurements. Alternatively, continuous monitoring of the pulmonary artery (mixed venous) oxygen saturation is clinically useful in these patients.[18] In patients with chronic heart failure, changes in the pulmonary artery oxygen saturation parallel

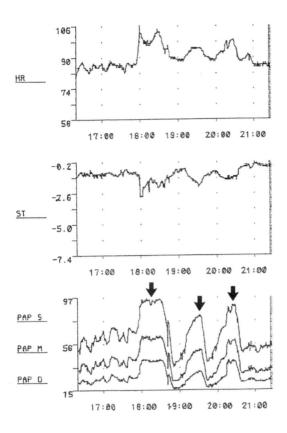

Figure 10.6 Dopamine induced myocardial ischemia in a woman with ischemic cardiomyopathy. Continuous recording of the heart rate (**HR**); the Lead II electrocardiographic ST segment (**ST**), and the pulmonary artery pressure (**PAP**) over 5 hours is shown. Dopamine therapy 3 µg/kg/min was begun to treat severe heart failure and is associated with the onset of episodes of acute myocardial ischemia (**arrows**). Each of the three episodes was stereotyped by tachycardia, ST segment depression, and profound pulmonary hypertension. At baseline, the heart rate is 85 beats/min and the pulmonary artery pressure is 59/24 mmHg. During peak ischemia, the heart rate is 103 beats/min, the pulmonary artery pressure is 96/43 mmHg and Lead II demonstrates 2.6 mm of ST segment depression. The episodes resolved when nitroprusside was substituted for dopamine.

HR = heart rate (scale is 58 to 106 beats/min); ST = ST segment (Scale is -7.4 to -0.2 mm); PAP = pulmonary artery pressure; S = systolic; M = mean; D = diastolic; Scale is 15 to 97 mmHg.

changes in the cardiac output.[16] Measurement of pulmonary artery oxygen saturation over time can be used to gauge the effects of therapy on the cardiac output *(Figure 10.5)*.[19]

Cautions

In some patients, aggressive medical management can worsen heart failure. This is especially true in patients with ischemic cardiomyopathy. Therapy with intravenous inotropic drugs or powerful vasodilator drugs can trigger episodes of myocardial ischemia thus worsening the heart failure. Careful examination of heart rate, pulmonary artery pressure, and wedge pressure data over time provides the astute clinician with the evidence that heart failure treatment may be harming the patient *(Figure 10.6)*.

This chapter has focused on the hemodynamic findings in patients with a dilated cardiomyopathy. The hemodynamic features of unusual heart diseases such as restrictive cardiomyopathy and "diastolic" heart failure are discussed in detail elsewhere[20-23] and in Chapter 12.

Key Points: Chronic Congestive Heart Failure

- The physical examination often seriously under-estimates the severity of the hemodynamic status of patients with chronic congestive heart failure.

- Intracardiac pressures are usually much higher than those observed during acute heart failure.

- The thermodilution method of cardiac output measurement may be inaccurate due to the presence of severe tricuspid regurgitation. Continuous measurement of the mixed venous oxygen saturation is a useful alternative.

- Aggressive therapy of chronic heart failure can aggravate myocardial ischemia.

Chapter 10 References

1. Stevenson LW, Perloff JK. The limited reliability of physical signs for estimating hemodynamics in chronic heart failure. *JAMA* 1989 261:884-888.

2. Butman SM, Ewy G, Standen JR, Kern KB, Hahn E. Bedside cardiovascular examination in patients with severe chronic heart failure: Importance of rest or inducible jugular venous distension. *J Am Coll Cardiol* 1993;22:968-74.

3. Chakko S, Woska D, Martinez H, DeMarchena E, Futterman L, Kessler KM, Myerburg RJ. Clinical, radiographic, and hemodynamic correlation's in chronic congestive heart failure: Conflicting results may lead to inappropriate care. *Am J Med* 1991;90:353-9.

4. Szidon JP, Pietra GG, Fishman AP. The alveolar-capillary membrane and pulmonary edema. *N Engl J Med* 1972;286:1200-4.

5. Staub NC, Nagano H, Pearce ML. Pulmonary edema in dogs, especially the sequence of fluid accumulation in lungs. *J Appl Physiol* 1967;22:227-40.

6. Dash H, Lipton MJ, Chatterjee K, Parmley WW. Estimation of pulmonary artery wedge pressure from chest radiograph in patients with chronic congestive cardiomyopathy and ischemic cardiomyopathy. *Br Heart J* 1980;44:322-9.

7. Coles NA, Hibberd M, Russell M, Love T, Ory D, Field TS, Dec GW, Eagle KA. Potential impact of pulmonary artery catheter placement on short-term management decisions in the medical intensive care unit. *Am Heart J* 1993;126:815-819.

8. Guila NH, Cohn JN, Mikulic E, Franciosa JA, Limas CJ. Treatment of refractory heart failure with infusion of nitroprusside. *N Engl J Med* 1974;291:587-592.

9. Stevenson LW, Dracrup KA, Tillisch JH. Efficacy of medical therapy tailored for severe congestive heart failure in patients transferred for urgent cardiac transplantation. *Am J Cardiol* 1989;63:461-464.

10. Forrester JS, Diamond G, Chatterjee K. Medical therapy of acute myocardial infarction by application of hemodynamic subsets. *N Engl J Med* 1976;295:1356-1362.

11. Hansing CE, Rowe GG. Tricuspid insufficiency. A study of hemodynamics and pathogenesis. *Circulation* 1972;45:793-799.

12. Kono T, Sabbah HN, Stein PD, Brymer JF, Khaja F. Left ventricular shape as a determinant of functional mitral regurgitation in patients with severe heart failure secondary to either coronary artery disease or idiopathic dilated cardiomyopathy. *Am J Cardiol* 1991;68:355-359.

13. Starr I. Clinical tests of the simple method of estimating cardiac stroke volume from blood pressure and age. *Circulation* 1954;9:664-681.

14. O'Rourke MF. The arterial pulse in health and disease. *Am Heart J* 1971;82:687-702.

15. Gleason WL, Braunwald E. Relationships between left ventricular end-diastolic volume and stroke volume in man with observations on the mechanism of pulsus alternans. *Circulation* 1962;25:841-848.

16. Finch CA, Lenfant C. Oxygen transport in man. *N Engl J Med* 1972;286:407-414.

17. Hamilton MA, Stevenson LW, Woo M, Child JS, Tillisch JH. Effect of tricuspid regurgitation on the reliability of the thermodilution cardiac output technique in congestive heart failure. *Am J Cardiol* 1989;64:945-948.

18. Divertie MB, McMichan JC. Continuous monitoring of mixed venous oxygen saturation. *Chest* 1984;85:423-428.

19. Gore JM, Sloan K. Use of continuous monitoring of mixed venous saturation in the Coronary Care Unit. *Chest* 1984;86:757-761.

20. Shabetai R, Fowler NO, Fenton JC. Restrictive cardiac disease: Pericarditis and the myocardiopathies. *Am Heart J* 1965;69:271-280.

21. Benotti JR, Grossman W, Cohn PF. Clinical profile of restrictive cardio-myopathy. *Circulation* 1980;61:1206-1212.

22. Schoenfeld MH, Supple EW, Dec GW Jr., Fallon JT, Palacios IF. Restrictive cardiomyopathy versus constrictive pericarditis: Role of endomyocardial biopsy in avoiding unnecessary thoracotomy. *Circulation* 1987;75:1012-1017.

23. Goldsmith SR, Dick C. Differentiating systolic from diastolic heart failure: Pathophysiologic and therapeutic considerations. *Am J Med* 1993;95:645-655.

PERICARDIAL TAMPONADE

C ardiac tamponade is an uncommon but life-threatening condition. The hemodynamic findings are fascinating. The astute clinician can establish the diagnosis of tamponade simply by a careful examination of the right atrial pressure waveform. Pericardial tamponade is a continuum with the degree of hemodynamic abnormality determined largely by the degree of fluid compression present.[1-2] The rate of pericardial fluid accumulation, the volume of fluid, the tensile properties of the pericardium, and the volume status of the patient are all variables which will affect the hemodynamic parameters.[3] The classic features of extreme cardiac tamponade include elevation and equalization of intracardiac pressures, pulsus paradoxus, and arterial hypotension.

Physiology of Tamponade

As fluid accumulates within the pericardial sac, the intrapericardial pressure rises.[1,3-5] Initially, the intrapericardial pressure is less than either the right atrial pressure or the wedge pressure.[1,3-5] At this stage, pulsus paradoxus is absent and the cardiac output is unchanged. As more fluid accumulates, the intrapericardial pressure rises to equal the right atrial pressure, but is still less

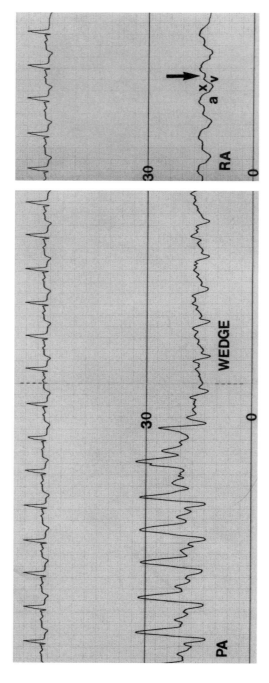

Figure 11.1 Pulmonary artery, wedge, and right atrial pressure waveforms from a patient with cardiac tamponade. Sinus rhythm is present. The pulmonary artery pressure is 31/13 mmHg; the mean wedge pressure is 15 mmHg; and the mean right atrial pressure is 13 mmHg. Note that the pulmonary artery diastolic pressure, the mean wedge pressure, and the mean right atrial pressure are essentially equal. The mean right atrial pressure is elevated with a prominent X descent (**x**) and an absent Y descent (**arrow**). This constellation of findings is highly specific for cardiac tamponade. Scale = 0–30 mmHg; Paper speed = 25 mm/sec.

than the wedge pressure.[1,3-5] Tamponade of the right heart now exists and the stroke volume is compromised.[1,3-5] Pulsus paradoxus may now appear.[1,3-5] With a further increase in the pericardial fluid, the intrapericardial pressure rises to the level of the wedge pressure.[1,3-5] Fluid compression of both the right and left heart now exists and the pericardial pressure, right atrial pressure, and wedge pressure are now equal.[1,3-5] Pulsus paradoxus is magnified and the stroke volume is significantly reduced.[1,3-5] Any additional accumulation of pericardial fluid further elevates both right atrial and wedge pressures equally and further compromises stroke volume until shock and death occur. Obviously, the rate of pericardial fluid accumulation will determine whether the physician is allowed to observe the hemodynamic features of each stage described above.

Right Atrial, Wedge, and Pulmonary Artery Pressures

The mean right atrial pressure is usually elevated with values of 10-15 mmHg commonly observed.[1,3-5] Patients with underlying heart disease may exhibit a higher mean right atrial pressure while patients with volume depletion may have a near normal right atrial pressure.[6] Cardiac tamponade alters the right atrial pressure waveform in a very helpful way: the X descent is prominent while the Y descent is markedly attenuated and often absent[3] *(Figures 11.1 & 11.2).* This important phenomenon can be explained as follows. During tamponade, the right atrial pressure is governed by the intrapericardial pressure. The intrapericardial pressure rises and falls during the cardiac cycle as the heart size increases and decreases. During ventricular systole, blood is ejected from the heart into the great vessels causing a decrease in the heart size and a decrease in the intrapericardial pressure. The right atrial pressure X descent (a ventricular systolic event) is thus magnified.

In contrast, the Y descent is either attenuated or absent. At the time of the Y descent, blood is transferred from the atria into the ventricles; the total cardiac volume is therefore unchanged.

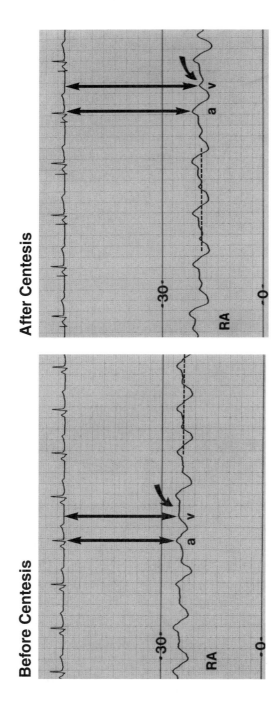

Figure 11.2 Right atrial pressure waveform from a patient with cardiac tamponade before (**left**) and after (**right**) pericardiocentesis. Sinus rhythm is present. During tamponade (**left**), the mean right atrial pressure is markedly elevated (23 mmHg). The X descent is prominent, but the Y descent is absent (**arrow**). After successful pericardiocentesis (**right**), the mean right atrial pressure has fallen (18 mmHg) and the Y descent has returned (**arrow**). The right atrial pressure remains elevated because of an underlying cardiomyopathy. Scale = 0-30 mmHg; Paper speed = 25 mm/sec.

Because the total cardiac volume is unchanged, the intrapericardial pressure does not change and the Y descent does not occur. With relief of the tamponade, the mean atrial pressure falls and Y descent reappears[3] *(Figure 11.2).* These fine details are best observed in the right atrial pressure waveform for two reasons. First, tamponade of the right heart usually precedes that of the left heart. Second, the right atrial pressure waveform is recorded directly from the proximal lumen and is not subject to the loss of fine detail caused by damping in the wedge pressure waveform.

Often, by the time cardiac tamponade is recognized, the intrapericardial pressure is already at the level of the mean wedge pressure. At this stage, equalization of the mean right atrial pressure and the mean wedge pressure is present *(Figure 11.1).* It is common to observe equalization of the mean right atrial pressure, the mean wedge pressure, and the pulmonary artery diastolic pressure because the pulmonary artery diastolic pressure is normally very close to the mean wedge pressure *(Figure 11.1).*

It is a common misconception that an inspiratory increase in the right atrial pressure (Kussmaul's sign) is present with pericardial tamponade.[7] In fact, Kussmaul's sign is observed in patients with pericardial constriction, not tamponade. In pure cardiac tamponade, the mean right atrial pressure falls slightly on inspiration.[3] Shabetai offers the following explanation for this observation: with pericardial constriction, the scarred pericardium effectively blocks the transmission of the inspiratory fall of intrathoracic pressure to the right atrium; with tamponade, the pericardial fluid allows the transmission of the inspiratory fall of intrathoracic pressure to the right atrium.[3]

Arterial Pressure

Alfred Kussmaul is responsible for describing pulsus paradoxus in patients with pericardial tamponade.[8] A widely accepted definition states that pulsus paradoxus exists when a normal inspiration is accompanied by a drop in the systolic arterial

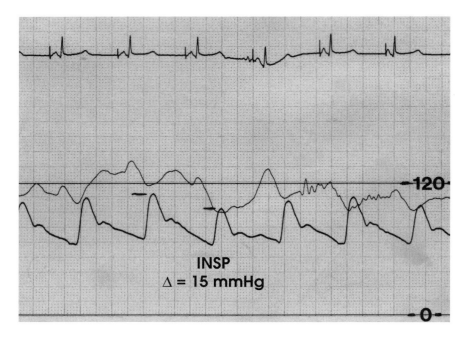

Figure 11.3 Simultaneous recording of arterial pressure and respiration from a patient with cardiac tamponade demonstrating pulsus paradoxus. On inspiration (**INSP**), the systolic arterial pressure declines by 15 mmHg. Note that the decline in the systolic arterial pressure is greater than the decline in the diastolic arterial pressure. As a result, the pulse pressure also declines on inspiration. Scale = 0-120 mmHg; Paper speed = 25 mm/sec.

pressure $\geq$ 10 mm.[3] This definition is somewhat arbitrary because the systolic pressure drops slightly on inspiration in normal individuals.[9] Pulsus paradoxus is a nonspecific finding and can be observed in patients with significant lung disease or shock.[10,11] With tamponade, the respiratory variation of the diastolic arterial pressure is less than that of the systolic pressure resulting in a significant inspiratory fall in the arterial pulse pressure[3] *(Figure 11.3)*. The magnitude of the inspiratory decrease in the arterial systolic pressure increases as the degree of tamponade increases.[12]

As pointed out by Shabetai, the use of the term "paradox" is misleading because it implies a response opposite to the normal.[3]

Pulsus paradoxus is actually an exaggeration of a normal finding. In Kussmaul's original description, the pulsus paradoxus was absolute (the peripheral pulse disappeared completely on inspiration).[3] Kussmaul's "paradox" was the auscultation of regular heart sounds accompanied by an irregular pulse.[3]

Pulsus paradoxus may be attenuated or absent in patients with cardiac tamponade and coexisting left ventricular dysfunction.[13] The mechanism for this observation is unclear but it is likely related to the "resistance" to compression of the left atrium afforded by an elevated left atrial pressure.[13]

Intuition might lead one to expect a low arterial pressure in patients with cardiac tamponade. This is true when the tamponade occurs abruptly. However, there is a distinct subgroup of patients with cardiac tamponade who present with hypertension rather than hypotension.[14] In this subgroup of patients, relief of the tamponade is associated with a decline in the arterial blood pressure.[14] These patients are more likely to have tamponade associated with a gradual fluid accumulation caused by conditions such as uremia or malignancy.[14]

Cardiac Output/Cardiac Index

In cardiac tamponade the cardiac index varies widely from normal to levels associated with shock because cardiac tamponade represents a spectrum of hemodynamic abnormalities.[1,3-5] Sinus tachycardia is a powerful compensatory response in these patients and tends to preserve the cardiac output/index. Measurement of the stroke volume is crucial.

Tamponade vs. Constriction

Patients with cardiac tamponade will commonly also have an inflamed and abnormal visceral and parietal pericardium. The hemodynamic findings of cardiac tamponade are present until the pericardial fluid is removed. At this time, the hemodynamic features of pericardial constriction become evident with a prominent right atrial pressure Y descent and appearance of Kussmaul's sign.[15] This syndrome is commonly referred to as effusive-constrictive pericarditis[15] and is discussed further in Chapter 12.

 ## Key Points: Pericardial Tamponade

- The mean right atrial pressure is elevated. The Y descent is attenuated or absent.

- With significant tamponade, the right atrial pressure, wedge pressure, and pulmonary artery diastolic pressure are usually equal.

- Pulsus paradoxus is present. The magnitude of the inspiratory decrease in arterial systolic pressure correlates with the degree of tamponade.

- An inspiratory increase in the right atrial pressure (Kussmaul's sign) is not observed in pure cardiac tamponade.

- Arterial hypertension can be observed despite significant tamponade.

Chapter 11 References

1. Reddy PS, Curtiss EI, Uretsky B. Spectrum of hemodynamic changes in cardiac tamponade. *Am J Cardiol* 1980;66:1487-1491.

2. Kern MJ, Aguirre FV. Pericardial compressive hemodynamics: Part I. In: Kern MJ, editor. *Hemodynamic Rounds: Interpretation of Cardiac Pathophysiology from Pressure Waveform Analysis.* New York: Wiley-Liss, 1993;83-89.

3. Shabetai R. *The Pericardium.* New York: Grune and Stratton, 1981; 224-324.

4. Reddy PS, Curtiss EI, O'Toole JD, Shaver JA. Cardiac tamponade: Hemodynamic observations in man. *Circulation* 1978;58:265-272.

5. Shabetai R, Fowler NO, Guntheroth WG. The hemodynamics of cardiac tamponade and constrictive pericarditis. *Am J Cardiol* 1970;26:480-489.

6. Antman EM, Cargill V, Grossman W. Low-pressure cardiac tamponade. *Ann Intern Med* 1979;91:403-406.

7. Spodick DH. Kussmaul's sign. *N Engl J Med* 1975;293:1047-8.

8. Kussmaul A. Ueber Schwieligie Mediastino: Pericarditis und den paradoxenpuls. *B Klin Wschr* 1873;10:433-435.

9. Shabetai R, Fowler NO, Gueron M. Effects of respiration on aortic pressure and flow. *Am Heart J* 1963;65:525-533.

10. McGregor M. Pulsus paradoxus. *N Engl J Med* 1979;301:480-482.

11. Cohn JN, Pinkerson AL, Tristani FE. Mechanism of pulsus paradoxus in clinical shock. *J Clin Invest* 1967;46:1744-1755.

12. Curtiss EI, Reddy PS, Uretsky BF, Cecchetti AA. Pulsus paradoxus: Definition and relation to the severity of cardiac tamponade. *Am Heart J* 1988;115:391-398.

13. Hoit BD, Gabel M, Fowler NO. Cardiac tamponade in left ventricular dysfunction. *Circulation* 1990; 82:1370-1376.

14. Brown J, McKinnon D, King A, Vanderbush E. Elevated arterial blood pressure in cardiac tamponade. *N Engl J Med* 1992;327:463-466.

15. Hancock EW. Subacute effusive constrictive pericarditis. *Circulation* 1971;43:183-192.

12

PERICARDIAL CONSTRICTION & RESTRICTIVE CARDIOMYOPATHY

A lthough pericardial constriction and restrictive cardiomyopathy are very different diseases, both share several clinical and hemodynamic features. With both constriction and restriction, the principle physiologic abnormality is impaired cardiac filling. In both conditions, the atrial pressures are elevated and the atrial pressure waveforms have steep X and Y descents.

With pericardial constriction, an unyielding pericardium is the culprit; with restrictive cardiomyopathy, the problem is an abnormal myocardium. In some patients, there is overlap between the two conditions. For example, with pericardial constriction, the inflammation may also invade the epicardium. Nonetheless, pericardial constriction can usually be differentiated from restrictive cardiomyopathy with careful attention to the hemodynamic findings.

Pericardial Constriction

Infection, inflammation, and neoplasm can each cause the pericardium to become thickened, scarred, and noncompliant. With constriction, the diastolic volume of the heart is reduced and the ventricular and atrial filling pressures are elevated. Since the

Figure 12.1 Right atrial (**RA**) and wedge pressure waveforms from a patient with pericardial constriction. The pressure waveforms are typical of constriction with a dominant Y descent (X < Y pattern). The mean RA pressure is 18 mmHg and the mean wedge pressure is 19 mmHg. Although the mean pressures are nearly equal, the A wave (**a**) in the wedge pressure waveform is more prominent than that in the RA tracing. Scale = 0-30 mmHg; Paper speed = 25 mm/sec.

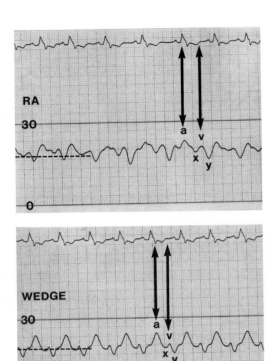

constricting process is usually uniform, all four cardiac chambers are involved equally (in contrast to restrictive cardiomyopathy). Right ventricular infarction mimics constriction because the sudden dilation of the right ventricle overdistends an otherwise normal pericardium (*Chapter 8*).

Intracardiac Pressures

The right atrial pressure and wedge pressure are significantly elevated. The magnitude of the atrial pressure elevation is determined by the degree of constriction.[1-4] With moderate constriction, the atrial pressures are between 12 and 15 mmHg; with severe constriction, the atrial pressures reach 20-25 mmHg. In pure constriction, the right atrial and wedge pressures are

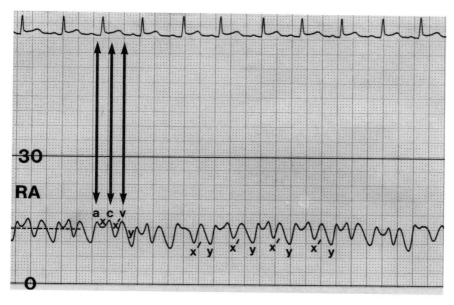

Figure 12.2 Right atrial (**RA**) pressure waveform typical of pericardial constriction. The mean right atrial pressure is elevated at 13 mmHg. The X'(**x'**) and Y (**y**) descents are both prominent with a pattern of X' < Y. The waveform resembles the letter W. This pattern can also occur with restrictive cardiomyopathy. Note that a well-developed C wave (**c**) interrupts the X descent (**x**) generating two components, the X and X′ descents. Scale = 0-30 mmHg; Paper speed = 25 mm/sec.

nearly identical *(Figure 12.1)*. However, coexisting mitral or tricuspid regurgitation can modify this relation. For example, if significant mitral regurgitation is present, the wedge pressure will significantly exceed the right atrial pressure.

In pericardial constriction, rapid filling of the ventricles is limited to early diastole (the ventricular size is smallest at the start of diastole, therefore, the ventricular constriction is least at this time). This exaggerated early ventricular filling results in a steep Y descent in the atrial pressure waveform.[1-4] Following atrial systole, the atrial volume is reduced (the atrial contents having been transported into the ventricles). At this time, constriction of the two atria transiently lessens resulting in a steep

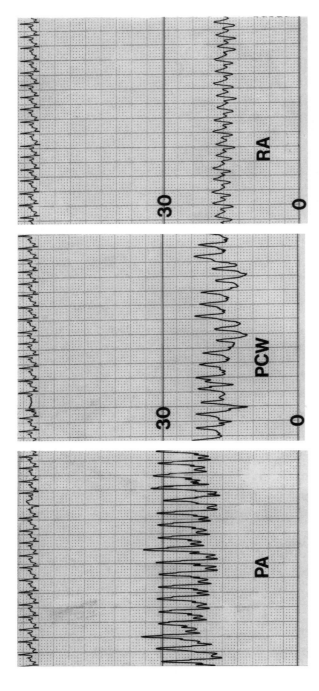

Figure 12.3 Pulmonary artery (**PA**), wedge (**PCW**), and right atrial (**RA**) pressure recordings from a patient with pericardial constriction. The pulmonary artery pressure is moderately elevated (32/19 mmHg). The mean wedge pressure is 17 mmHg while the mean right atrial pressure is 16 mmHg. Although the mean atrial pressures are nearly equal, the waveforms are not identical. Note the absence of respiratory variation in the right atrial pressure tracing (in constriction, absence of respiratory variation is more common than is Kussmaul's sign). Scale = 0-30 mmHg; Paper speed = 6.25 mm/sec.

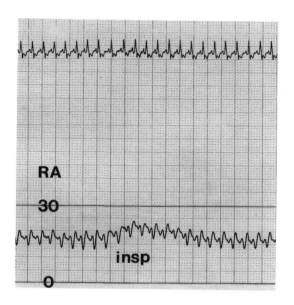

Figure 12.4 Right atrial (**RA**) pressure tracing from a patient with severe pericardial constriction. With inspiration (**insp**), the mean right atrial pressure increases (Kussmaul's sign). Scale = 0-30 mmHg; Paper speed = 6.25 mm/sec.

X descent.[1-4] The combination of a steep X and steep Y descent causes the atrial pressure waveform to resemble the letter W (or M depending on your preference, *Figures 12.1 & 12.2).* This pattern can be observed in conditions other than pericardial constriction. In patients with constriction, atrial fibrillation is common and will cause the A wave to disappear from the pressure waveform.

The presence of a noncompliant pericardium limits the transmission of intrathoracic pressure to the heart.[1] The normal inspiratory increase in superior and inferior vena cava flow is reduced or absent.[1,2] Therefore, the right atrial pressure often shows no respiratory change[1,2] *(Figure 12.3).* With severe constriction, an inspiratory increase in the right atrial pressure (Kussmaul's sign) may be present, but this is the exception, not the rule[1,2] *(Figure 12.4).*

In pericardial constriction the pulmonary artery pressure is modestly elevated. The pulmonary artery systolic pressure is typically 35-45 mmHg[1,2] *(Figure 12.3)*. Severe pulmonary hypertension suggests coexisting myocardial or valvular heart disease. The pulmonary artery diastolic pressure should equal both the right atrial pressure and the wedge pressure *(Figure 12.3)*.

In pericardial constriction the aortic pressure is usually maintained. Pulsus paradoxus is observed in only about one-third of patients with pericardial constriction, whereas in pericardial tamponade pulsus paradoxus is nearly universal.[1-3] The stroke volume is reduced but tachycardia can maintain the cardiac output in all but the most severe cases. With severe constriction the stroke volume index may be as low as 15-25 mL/m[2]. [1,2]

Effusive-Constrictive Pericarditis

In some patients, pericardial inflammation leads to the combination of a pericardial effusion and pericardial constriction. In effusive-constrictive pericarditis, there is constriction of the heart by the visceral pericardium and pericardial fluid accumulation between the visceral and parietal pericardium.[5] Tuberculosis, mediastinal radiation, uremia, and pericardial malignancy are conditions known to cause effusive-constrictive pericarditis.[1,2,6]

Hemodynamic Findings

The characteristic hemodynamic findings of effusive-constrictive pericarditis were first reported by Hancock.[7] The hemodynamic findings of pericardial tamponade dominate until removal of the pericardial effusion at which time the findings of constriction becomes apparent.

With effusive-constrictive pericarditis the right atrial and wedge pressures are elevated and equalized. The mean right atrial pressure is typically 11-25 mmHg (average 18 mmHg).[2,7] Prior to pericardiocentesis, the atrial pressure waveform resembles pericardial tamponade with a prominent X descent and an attenuated or absent Y descent *(Figure 12.5)*. An inspiratory increase in the mean right atrial pressure

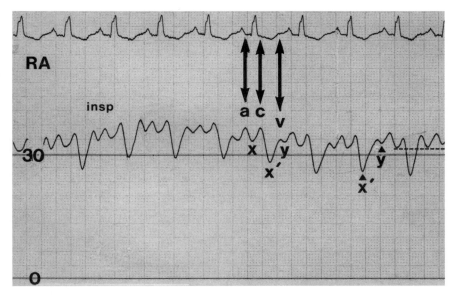

Figure 12.5 Right atrial (**RA**) pressure tracing from a patient with uremia and effusive-constrictive pericarditis. The mean right atrial pressure is markedly elevated at 31 mmHg. The X descent (**x**)is dominant (X > Y pattern). The Y descent (**y**) is attenuated due to the presence of pericardial fluid compression. On inspiration (**insp**), the mean right atrial pressure rises (Kussmaul's sign). Scale = 0-30 mmHg; Paper speed = 25 mm/sec.

(Kussmaul's sign) is rare and usually present only with severe effusive-constrictive pericarditis *(Figure 12.5).*[6] Prior to pericardiocentesis, pulsus paradoxus may be present (one-third of cases) which disappears after removal of the fluid. The diagnosis of effusive-constrictive pericarditis is best made when careful hemodynamic monitoring is performed during and after pericardiocentesis.

After pericardiocentesis, the atrial pressure waveform is converted to that of constriction with the appearance of a steep Y descent (X = Y or X < Y).[2,7] After removal of the pericardial fluid, the right atrial and wedge pressures fall modestly (5 mmHg on average). The atrial pressures remain elevated due to the presence of constriction. Prior to pericardiocentesis, the right atrial pressure does not decrease with inspiration (with pure tamponade, the mean right atrial pressure normally falls with inspiration).[3,7]

Restrictive Cardiomyopathy

Restrictive cardiomyopathy is a myocardial disease. Myocardial relaxation is restricted resulting in a hemodynamic picture closely resembling pericardial constriction. Restrictive cardiomyopathy is uncommon. Its causes include rather obscure diseases such as hemochromatosis, endomyocardial fibrosis, amyloidosis, and myocarditis.

Hemodynamic Findings

With restrictive cardiomyopathy the right atrial pressure and wedge pressures are significantly elevated to levels observed with pericardial constriction (15-25 mmHg).[2,8,9] As with constriction, the X and Y descents are prominent with a pattern of X = Y or Y > X. In contrast to constrictive pericarditis, the right atrial pressure and wedge pressure are usually not equal. The restrictive process involves both the left and right ventricle and causes a proportionate decrease in each chamber's distensibility. As a result, the left and right ventricular filling pressures are elevated but not equal. The wedge pressure usually exceeds the right atrial pressure.[9] The difference between the wedge pressure and the right atrial pressure may be only a few millimeters of mercury; a difference that can be difficult to precisely measure at the bedside. Certain maneuvers can be used in an attempt to further diverge the right and left ventricular filling pressures. These include exercise, induced premature ventricular beats, and the Valsalva maneuver.[2] These are best performed in the cardiac catheterization laboratory during high fidelity recordings of the right and left ventricular diastolic pressures.

Pulmonary hypertension is often more severe in restrictive cardiomyopathy than in constrictive pericarditis.[2] In restriction, the pulmonary artery systolic pressure typically exceeds 50 mmHg; in

PERICARDIAL CONSTRICTION

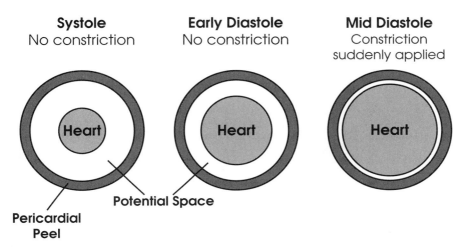

Systole	**Early Diastole**	**Mid Diastole**
No constriction	No constriction	Constriction suddenly applied

Potential Space

Pericardial Peel

Figure 12.6 Schematic demonstrating the effect of pericardial constriction on the heart. During ventricular systole (**left**) constriction is absent. The systolic venous return to the atria (X descent) is unimpaired. During early ventricular diastole (**middle**) constriction is still absent. The initial Y descent is unimpaired. In mid diastole (**right**), the heart volume suddenly equals the pericardial volume and constriction occurs. Diastolic filling is abruptly halted resulting in an abrupt halt to the Y descent. Adapted from Shabetai, R.[1]

constriction this level of pulmonary hypertension is unusual.[2] Pulsus paradoxus can be observed in restriction but is uncommon.[2] The cardiac index may be normal but maintained by tachycardia.[9]

Conclusion

The hemodynamic findings of pericardial constriction, effusive constrictive pericarditis, pericardial tamponade, and restrictive cardiomyopathy are compared in *Table 12.1* and *Figure 12.6 & 12.7*. The term "constrictive physiology" describes the hemodynamic condition of elevated atrial pressures with steep X and Y descents in the atrial pressure waveform. These hemodynamic findings can be caused by either constrictive pericarditis or restrictive cardiomyopathy. Differentiating the two may be difficult or even impossible using bedside hemodynamic measurements. The

PERICARDIAL TAMPONADE

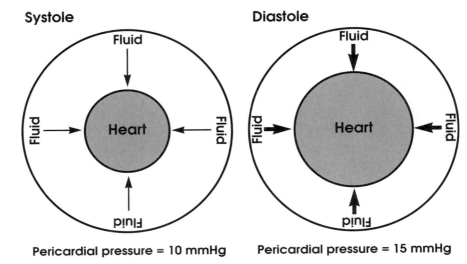

Figure 12.7 Schematic demonstrating the effect of pericardial tamponade on the heart. The atrial pressures are governed by the elevated pericardial pressure. During early ventricular systole (**left**) the total heart size decreases as blood is ejected from the ventricles. Consequently, the pericardial pressure drops transiently resulting in an X descent in the atrial pressure waveform. During late systole, the heart size has started to increase because of venous return to the atria resulting in a progressive increase in the pericardial pressure. During early diastole (**right**) blood is transferred from the atria to the ventricles. The total cardiac volume remains constant and therefore the pericardial pressure also remains constant. The result is an absent Y descent. Adapted from Shabetai, R.[1]

presence of atrial fibrillation or valvular insufficiency (mitral or tricuspid) can further complicate the hemodynamic findings. Establishing the correct diagnosis is crucial because treatment of the two conditions is radically different. When uncertainty persists despite careful bedside hemodynamic measurements, formal cardiac catheterization is essential. Doppler echocardiography, radionuclide angiography, and computerized tomography or magnetic resonance imaging have proven useful in some patients.[10] In the exceptional case, an exploratory thoracotomy to examine the pericardium may be required.[9]

Table 12.1	Comparison of Typical Hemodynamic Findings in Pericardial Constriction, Effusive-Constrictive Pericarditis, Restrictive Cardiomyopathy & Pericardial Tamponade			
	Tamponade	Constriction	Effusive-Constrictive	Restriction
RA Pressure Mean Range (mmHg)	15 10-25	15 10-25	18 10-30	15 10-25
RA Waveform	X > Y (Y often absent)	X = Y or X < Y	X > Y (pre-tap) X = Y or X < Y (post-tap)	X = Y or X < Y
RA/Wedge Relation	Equal	Equal	Equal	Wedge > RA
PA Systolic Pressure	Normal or minimally elevated	35-40 mmHg	Similar to constriction	Often >50 mmHg
Kussmaul's Sign	Absent (RA pressure falls with inspiration)	Present in 1/3 of cases (especially with severe constriction)	Rare unless severe	May be present
Pulsus Paradoxus	Almost always	Present in 1/3	present - pre-tap absent - post-tap	Uncommon

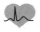 ### Key Points: Pericardial Constriction & Restrictive Cardiomyopathy

- Pericardial constriction and restrictive cardiomyopathy share many common features. Cardiac filling is abnormal in both conditions.

- The right atrial pressure and the wedge pressure are elevated in both conditions. The degree of pressure elevation in the atria parallels the severity of the constriction/restriction.

- With pure pericardial constriction the right atrial pressure and wedge pressure are nearly equal (within 5 mmHg).

- With restrictive cardiomyopathy the right atrial pressure and the wedge pressure are often dissociated by ≥ 5 mmHg.

- Pulmonary hypertension is usually more severe with restrictive cardiomyopathy. The pulmonary artery systolic pressure usually exceeds 50 mmHg.

- Atrial fibrillation and/or mitral/tricuspid valve regurgitation are common complications of both conditions. Either the abnormal rhythm or the valvular regurgitation can further alter the hemodynamic findings.

- Pericardial effusion can coexist with pericardial constriction creating a unique hemodynamic condition known as effusive-constrictive pericarditis.

- In some patients it is not possible to differentiate pericardial constriction from restrictive cardiomyopathy using hemodynamic measurements.

Chapter 12 References

1. Shabetai R. *The Pericardium.* New York: Grune & Stratton,1981:154-223.

2. Shabetai R, Grossman W. Profiles in constrictive pericarditis, restrictive cardiomyopathy, and cardiac tamponade. In: Grossman W. *Cardiac Catheterization and Angiography,* 2nd ed. Philadelphia: Lea & Febiger, 1980:358-376.

3. Shabetai R, Fowler NO, Guntheroth WG. The hemodynamics of cardiac tamponade and contrictive pericarditis. *Am J Cardiol* 1970;26:480-489.

4. Hansen AT, Eskildsen P, Gotzsche H. Pressure curves from the right auricle and right ventricle in constrictive pericarditis. *Circulation* 1951;3:881-888.

5. Spodick DH, Kumar S. Subacute constrictive pericarditis with cardiac tamponade. *Dis Chest* 1968;54:62-66.

6. Mann T, Brodie BR, Grossman W, McLaurin LP. Effusive-constrictive hemodynamic pattern due to neoplastic involvement of the pericardium. *Am J Cardiol* 1978;41:781-786.

7. Hancock EW. Subacute effusive-constrictive pericarditis. *Circulation* 1971;43:183-192.

8. Meaney E, Shabetai R, Bhargava V, Shearer M, Weidner C, Mangiardi LM, Smalling R, Peterson K. Cardiac amyloidosis, constrictive pericarditis, and restrictive cardiomyopathy. *Am J Cardiol* 1976;38:547-556.

9. Benotti JR, Grossman W, Cohn PF. The clinical profile of restrictive cardiomyopathy. *Circulation* 1980;61:1206-1212.

10. Aroney CN, Ruddy TD, Dighero H, Fifer MA, Boucher CA, Palacios IF. Differentiation of restrictive cardiomyopathy from pericardial constriction: assessment of diastolic function by radionuclide angiography. *J Am Coll Cardiol* 1989;13:1007-1014.

13

PULMONARY EMBOLISM

B edside hemodynamic monitoring is rarely used to establish the diagnosis of pulmonary embolism. Nevertheless, the clinician must be familiar with the hemodynamic findings of pulmonary embolism because it is such a common complication of other serious illnesses in hospitalized patients. The hemodynamic findings observed with pulmonary embolism are due to an increase in the pulmonary vascular resistance. Acute pulmonary embolism has hemodynamic features which are different from those observed with chronic embolism.

Pulmonary Artery, Wedge, Right Atrial Pressures & Cardiac Output

Acute Pulmonary Embolism

Sinus tachycardia is the rule. Pulmonary hypertension is present in approximately 70% of patients.[1] In patients without prior cardiopulmonary disease, the mean pulmonary artery pressure is consistently increased when obstruction of the pulmonary vasculature exceeds 25-30%.[1] The mean pulmonary artery pressure usually does not exceed 40 mmHg because the normal right ventricle cannot generate a high pulmonary artery pressure acutely (*Figure 13.1*).[1] Higher levels of pulmonary artery pressure suggest a chronic component to the pulmonary embolism or pre-

Figure 13.1 Pulmonary artery (**PA**), wedge (**PCW**), and right atrial (**RA**) pressure waveforms from a patient with massive acute pulmonary embolism and shock. Sinus tachycardia (108 beats/min) is present. Modest pulmonary hypertension (42/24; mean 27 mmHg) is present. A significant pressure gradient between the pulmonary artery diastolic pressure (24 mmHg) and the mean wedge pressure (12 mmHg) is present reflecting an increased pulmonary vascular resistance. The elevated mean right atrial pressure (14 mmHg) signifies acute right heart failure. The ratio of mean right atrial pressure/mean wedge pressure (1.2) is increased. Scale = 0-25 mmHg; Paper speed = 10 mm/sec.

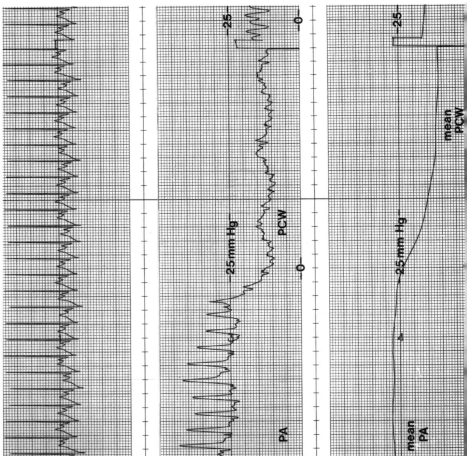

existing heart disease. The mean pulmonary artery pressure correlates well with the degree of angiographic obstruction.[1] With massive embolism, pulmonary artery pulsus alternans may appear.[2]

The mean wedge pressure is usually normal or low unless the patient has underlying heart disease.[3] When there is an obstruction in the pulmonary vasculature, a gradient between the pulmonary artery diastolic pressure and the mean wedge pressure is generated and the left atrial A and V waves are not transmitted retrogradely into the wedge pressure waveform (*Figures 13.1 & 13.2*).[3,4] There is concern that the wedge pressure may not reliably reflect the left atrial pressure in the presence of acute pulmonary embolism.[4,5] The mean wedge pressure should be interpreted cautiously in these patients.

The mean right atrial pressure is an important indicator of right ventricular function in acute pulmonary embolism.[1] The mean right atrial pressure increases in direct response to an increase in the pulmonary artery pressure.[1] An elevation of the mean right atrial pressure in a previously healthy patient usually indicates severe embolism with mean pulmonary artery pressures ≥ 30 mmHg and angiographic obstruction exceeding 35-40%[1] (*Figure 13.1*). On the other hand, significant angiographic obstruction (up to 40%) may occur without elevation of the mean right atrial pressure.[1] The right atrial A wave is often prominent in response to the sudden elevation of right ventricular diastolic pressure.[3] Tricuspid regurgitation may appear in response to right ventricular dilatation.

The pulmonary artery pressure and the mean right atrial pressure typically remain elevated for days after an acute pulmonary embolus.[7] At 2-3 weeks, the mean pulmonary artery pressure has frequently returned to normal, although persistent pulmonary hypertension occurs in some patients.[7]

With moderate embolism, the cardiac index is increased due in large part to an increase in both the stroke volume and the

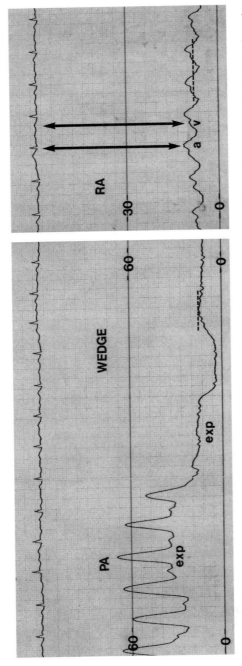

Figure 13.2 Pulmonary artery (**PA**), wedge, and right atrial (**RA**) pressure waveforms from a patient with chronic pulmonary embolism. The rhythm is sinus (95 beats/min). Significant pulmonary hypertension (67/33; mean 45 mmHg) is present. The gradient between the pulmonary artery diastolic pressure (33 mmHg) and the mean wedge pressure (16 mmHg) is markedly increased. The abnormal pulmonary vasculature prevents retrograde transmission of the left atrial A and V waves into the wedge pressure waveform. The mean right atrial pressure (8 mmHg) is mildly elevated signifying early right heart failure. The right atrial pressure A wave (**a**) is prominent reflecting more forceful right atrial contraction. Scale = 0-60 mmHg (PA and wedge) and 0-30 mmHg (RA). Paper speed = 25 mm/sec.

heart rate from endogenous catecholamine release.[1] With severe embolism and right heart failure, the cardiac index and stroke volume may be low and shock may occur.

Chronic Pulmonary Embolism

Pulmonary embolism sometimes leads to chronic pulmonary hypertension.[8-10] In chronic embolism, the pulmonary artery pressure is much higher than that observed during acute pulmonary embolism because the right ventricle has had the opportunity to hypertrophy in response to the pressure overload.[8-10] Pulmonary artery pressures at or above systemic arterial pressures are recorded in some of these patients. Because of the abnormal pulmonary vasculature, a significant gradient exists between the pulmonary artery diastolic pressure and the mean wedge pressure *(Figure 13.2)*. As with acute embolism, the left atrial A and V waves are not transmitted into the wedge pressure waveform and the mean wedge pressure may not be an accurate reflection of the true left atrial pressure *(Figure 13.2)*. Prolonged pulmonary hypertension usually leads to right heart failure with attendant elevation of the mean right atrial pressure. The right atrial pressure A wave is accentuated because of the noncompliant right ventricle *(Figure 13.2)*. With right ventricular failure, tricuspid regurgitation appears resulting in a prominent CV wave and Y descent in the right atrial pressure waveform *(Chapter 6)*. The right atrial pressure may exceed the left atrial pressure leading to a small right to left atrial shunt in those patients with a patent foramen ovale.[3]

The cardiac output/index is usually maintained until the late stages. The systemic arterial pressure is also normal. The systemic circulation is much more responsive to vasodilation than the pulmonary circulation and vasodilator drugs can cause serious hypotension in these patients.[11]

Cautions

Balloon inflation time should be kept to a minimum in patients with significant pulmonary hypertension because of an increased risk for pulmonary artery rupture.[12] Care should be used when inserting a pulmonary artery catheter into a patient with suspected pulmonary embolism because peripheral venous emboli can become trapped within the right atrium or right ventricle on their journey through the heart.[13] Insertion of the catheter can dislodge these clots with fatal consequences. In patients with suspected pulmonary embolism, a two-dimensional echocardiogram prior to catheter insertion can alert the physician to the presence of entrapped right heart clots.

Since pulmonary embolism is frequently a complication of other serious illnesses, the hemodynamic abnormalities observed may reflect a combination of several processes. This is especially likely in patients with chronic congestive heart failure *(Chapter 10)*. The observant clinician will consider pulmonary embolism whenever a gradient ≥ 5 mmHg exists between the pulmonary artery diastolic pressure and the mean wedge pressure.

 Key Points: Acute & Chronic Pulmonary Embolism

- In both acute and chronic pulmonary embolism, an increase in pulmonary vascular resistance leads to pulmonary hypertension.

- With acute pulmonary embolism, an elevated mean right atrial pressure suggests severe embolism. Elevation of the right atrial pressure is associated with a mean pulmonary artery pressure ≥ 30 mmHg and angiographic obstruction exceeding 35-40% of the pulmonary vascular bed.

- With both acute and chronic embolism, the pulmonary artery diastolic pressure is significantly higher than the mean wedge pressure. Distinct A and V waves are absent from the wedge pressure waveform. The mean wedge pressure may no longer be an accurate measure of the mean left atrial pressure.

- With both acute and chronic embolism, the right atrial pressure may exceed the left atrial pressure leading to a right to left shunt across a patent foramen ovale.

- Patients with pulmonary hypertension are at increased risk of pulmonary artery rupture during balloon inflation.

Chapter 13 References

1. McIntyre KM, Sasahara AA. The hemodynamic response to pulmonary embolism in patients without prior cardiopulmonary disease. *Am J Cardiol* 1971;28:288-294.

2. Calick A, Berger S. Pulmonary artery pulsus alternans associated with pulmonary embolism. *Chest* 1973;64:663.

3. Grossman W, Braunwald E. Pulmonary hypertension. In: Braunwald E, editor. *Heart Disease: A Textbook of Cardiovascular Medicine*, 3rd ed. Philadelphia: WB Saunders, 1988;811.

4. Jenkins BS, Bradley RD, Branthwaite MA. Evaluation of pulmonary arterial end-diastolic pressure is an indirect estimate of left atrial mean pressure. *Circulation* 1970;42:75-78.

5. Shaffer AB, Silber EN. Factors influencing the character of the pulmonary arterial wedge pressure. *Am Heart J* 1956;51:522-532.

6. Ankeney JL. Further experimental evidence that pulmonary capillary pressures do not reflect cyclic changes in left atrial pressure (mitral lesions and pulmonary embolism). *Circ Research* 1953;1:58-61.

7. Dalen JE, Banas JS, Brooks HL, Evans GL, Paraskos JA, Dexter L. Resolution rate of acute pulmonary embolism in man. *N Engl J Med* 1969;280:1194-1199.

8. Rich S, Levitsky S, Brundage BH. Pulmonary hypertension from chronic pulmonary thromboembolism. *Ann Int Med* 1988;108:425-434.

9. National Cooperative Study. The urokinase pulmonary embolism trial. *Circulation* 1973;47 (Suppl II):51-59.

10. Paraskos JA, Adelstein SJ, Smith RE, Rickman ED, Grossman W, Dexter L, Dalen JE. Late prognosis of acute pulmonary embolism. *N Engl J Med* 1973;289:55-58.

11. Packer M. Vasodilator therapy for primary pulmonary hypertension. Limitations and hazards. *Ann Intern Med* 1985;103:258-270.

12. Barash PG, Nardi D, Hammond G. Catheter-induced pulmonary artery perforation - mechanisms, management and modification. *J Thorac Cardiovasc Surg* 1981;82:5-12.

13. Saner HE, Asinger RW, Daniel JA, Elsperger KJ. Two-dimensional echocardiographic detection of right-sided cardiac intracavitary thromboembolus with pulmonary embolus. *J Am Coll Cardiol* 1984;4:1294-1301.

14

TROUBLE

Any physician who has used the pulmonary artery catheter extensively knows the meaning of the word trouble. An impressive list of problems can arise with the use of the pulmonary artery catheter.[1,2] Instead of restating these complications, this chapter will focus on selected common problems encountered during 13 years of hemodynamic monitoring in a coronary care unit. Some of the errors illustrated in this chapter may seem quite basic. Nonetheless, all were made by physicians or nursing staff familiar with the use of the pulmonary artery catheter.

Misinterpretation of the Wedge Pressure Waveform

Misinterpretation of the wedge pressure waveform is common and can lead to major errors in patient management.[3] When balloon inflation "wedges" the catheter, the pressure waveform suddenly changes. As a result, many physicians have learned to watch for a change in the pulmonary artery pressure waveform during balloon inflation and to automatically identify this new waveform as the wedge pressure. The pressure waveform itself may receive only a cursory glance. Although this process will be correct in most patients, occasionally a serious error will occur. For example, fluoroscopy reveals that the pulmonary artery

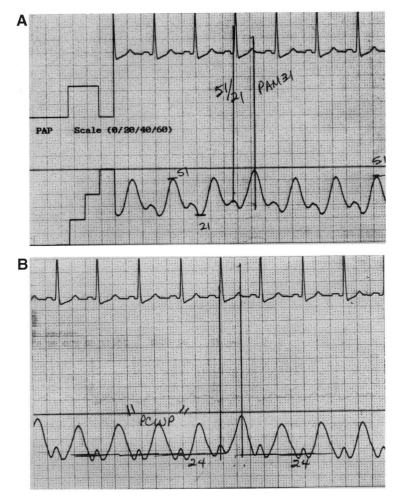

Figure 14.1 Incorrect interpretation of pressure waveforms. **Panel A:** The pulmonary artery pressure (PA) is recorded. **Panel B:** With balloon inflation, the waveform changes slightly. The tracing at bottom was interpreted as a wedge tracing (PCWP) with a mean wedge pressure of 35 mmHg and a large V-wave. In fact, the peak of this "V wave" occurs within the electrocardiographic T-wave, identical to the timing of the pulmonary artery systolic wave at top. The pressure tracing at bottom is therefore still pulmonary artery. The mean wedge pressure was actually only 20 mmHg. Scale = 0-60 mmHg; Paper speed = 25 mm/sec.

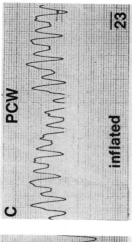
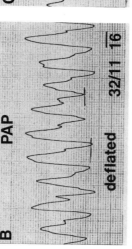
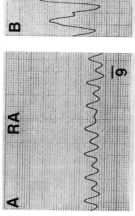

Figure 14.2 Incorrect interpretation of hemodynamic pressure waveforms. Panel A is the right atrial pressure waveform. Panel B was interpreted as the pulmonary artery pressure while Panel C was interpreted as the wedge pressure. The error was caused by improper catheter position (in this case the distal lumen was in the right ventricular outflow tract). With the balloon deflated (Panel B) during systole, the catheter tip moves into the proximal pulmonary artery (recording pulmonary artery systolic pressure and the dicrotic notch). During diastole, the catheter tip moves back into the right ventricle and records right ventricular diastolic pressure. With the balloon inflated (Panel C), the catheter tip remains in the pulmonary artery during both systole and diastole. Panel C is thus the pulmonary artery pressure waveform. Clues to the error include the fact that the diastolic pressure in Panel C is equal to the mean right atrial pressure (Panel A). Also, the mean pressure in Panel C is greater than the mean pressure in Panel B. The mean wedge pressure should never exceed the mean pulmonary artery pressure.
Scale = 0-40 mmHg; Paper speed = 25 mm/sec.

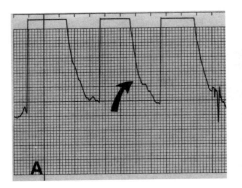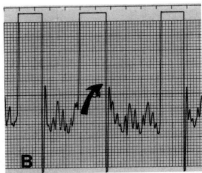

Figure 14.3 Abnormal (**Panel A**) and normal (**Panel B**) fast flush tests. In Panel A, the pressure decay (**arrow**) is gradual and smooth due to damping by an air bubble in the transducer dome. After removal of the air bubble (**Panel B**), the pressure decay (**arrow**) is very sharp and followed by a series of oscillations reflecting a highly responsive system.

catheter usually moves considerably with balloon inflation and that the catheter does not always "wedge" itself. This movement may change the pulmonary artery pressure waveform somewhat (sometimes referred to as a "partial wedge"). If this altered pulmonary artery pressure waveform is interpreted as the wedge pressure, serious errors in patient management will result *(Figure 14.1)*.

Positioning the distal lumen of the pulmonary artery catheter in the right ventricular outflow tract may cause a similar problem. With the balloon deflated, the catheter moves into the pulmonary artery during systole and into the right ventricle during diastole. With balloon inflation, the pressure waveform changes as the catheter moves into the pulmonary artery and remains there in both systole and diastole *(Figure 14.2)*. This new waveform can be mistakenly interpreted as the wedge pressure *(Figure 14.2)*. These and related errors can be avoided if the wedge pressure waveform is carefully analyzed, a process that usually requires less than one minute.

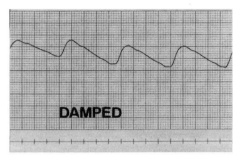

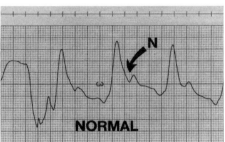

Figure 14.4 Damped pressure waveform. At top, the pulmonary artery pressure waveform is smooth with loss of fine detail due to a catheter kink. At bottom, with removal of the kink, the fine detail of the pressure waveform reappears. Note the dicrotic notch (**N**) has returned.

Damped Pressure Waveform

The pressure waveforms recorded with bedside equipment are prone to signal degradation by damping. This problem can be recognized prior to catheter insertion using the "fast flush" test[4] *(Figure 14.3)*. Damping causes a loss of fine detail in the pressure tracing resulting in a "smoothed" pressure tracing *(Figure 14.4)*. Disappearance of the dicrotic notch on the pulmonary artery pressure waveform is a helpful marker of a damped tracing *(Figure 14.4)*. The most common causes of a damped tracing (working from the distal catheter lumen backward) include: thrombus in the distal lumen; catheter kink (especially at the clavicle with subclavian insertion sites); air in the stopcocks or pressure transducer; and faulty transducer. Usually, flushing the system and purging the air will improve a damped tracing. The chest x-ray should be examined for a catheter kink near the introducer site. If these efforts fail, a new transducer and cable should be requested.

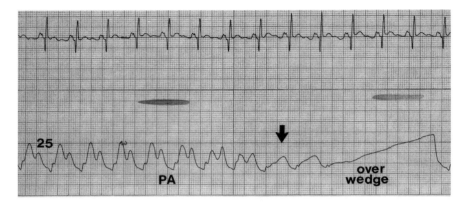

Figure 14.5 The "overwedge" tracing. Balloon inflation (**arrow**) yields a pressure tracing which continues to rise eventually exceeding the limits of the scale. In this patient, the pulmonary artery catheter is positioned too distal in the pulmonary artery. Balloon inflation causes the distal lumen to impact the pulmonary artery intima and occludes the distal lumen. The pressure within the distal lumen begins to rise because the catheter is being continuously flushed at a rate of 3 mL/hour and the pressure will eventually reach 300 mmHg (the pressure usually used to continuously flush the catheter). This "overwedge" waveform will therefore be observed whenever the distal lumen impacts vascular endothelium and is completely occluded. These patients are at risk for vascular perforation.
Scale = 0-25 mmHg; Paper speed = 25 mm/sec.

Overwedge

The term "overwedge" loosely refers to a pressure tracing which continues to rise until it disappears from the scale *(Figure 14.5)*. This pressure tracing occurs whenever the distal lumen is physically obstructed. The most common cause of obstruction is impact of the catheter tip against the intima of a blood vessel.

To maintain catheter patency, the distal lumen is continuously infused with heparinized solution at a rate of 3 mL/hour. The infused solution is usually pressurized to 250-300 mmHg. With distal lumen obstruction, the recorded pressure will eventually rise to this level. In practice, this "overwedge" tracing is most often encountered during balloon inflation when the catheter tip is located too far distally in the pulmonary vasculature. Inflation

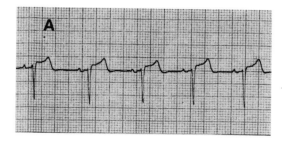

Figure 14.6 Right bundle branch block caused by pulmonary artery catheter insertion.
Panel A: Electrocardiographic Lead V_1 at baseline.

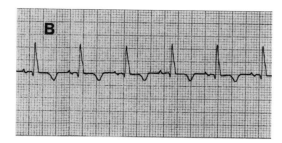

Panel B: Electrocardiographic Lead V_1 during catheter insertion demonstrates a typical right bundle branch block configuration. The electrocardiographic change was noticed retrospectively by the nursing staff.

of the balloon in an undersized pulmonary artery segment forces the catheter tip into the vessel intima and places the patient at risk for pulmonary artery perforation.[5,6] Whenever the "overwedge" tracing appears, the operator should assume that the catheter tip is against the vascular intima. The catheter should be repositioned immediately.

Arrhythmias

A variety of ventricular and supraventricular arrhythmias are caused by catheter contact with the right atrium or the right ventricle.[7] Catheter impact with the right side of the ventricular septum can cause right bundle branch block.[8] The operator is often unaware of the right bundle branch block because the QRS complex change may be subtle and because attention is usually focused on the pressure waveform and not the electrocardiogram *(Figure 14.6)*. Most often it is noticed by the nursing staff. Catheter induced right bundle branch block is usually transient and of no clinical consequence unless the patient has a pre-existing left bundle branch block. The outcome will then be

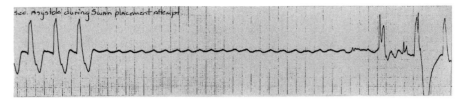

Figure 14.7 Transient complete heart block and asystole caused by pulmonary artery catheter insertion. The patient has an underlying complete left bundle branch block. Heart block resulted when the pulmonary artery catheter impacted against the septum causing a right bundle branch block. The underlying rhythm is atrial flutter.

complete heart block *(Figure 14.7)*. It is wise to be prepared for complete heart block with a standby external pacemaker when inserting a pulmonary artery catheter into a patient with left bundle branch block.

Cardiac Output

Naturally, errors can also occur during the measurement of the thermodilution cardiac output. An arrhythmia during the injection and recording of the thermodilution curve will yield a cardiac output measurement which is not representative of the patient's steady state *(Figure 14.8)*. These curves should be rejected. Examination of the thermodilution curve is a helpful exercise and occasionally produces an educational experience *(Figure 14.9)*.

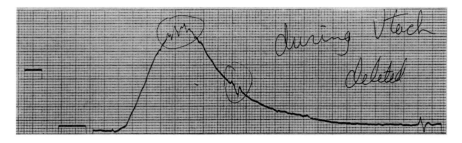

Figure 14.8 Arrhythmia during cardiac output measurement. This patient developed nonsustained ventricular tachycardia (**V tach**) during the recording of the thermodilution curve. This caused distortion of the curve (**circled areas**). This measurement was therefore rejected by the nursing staff.

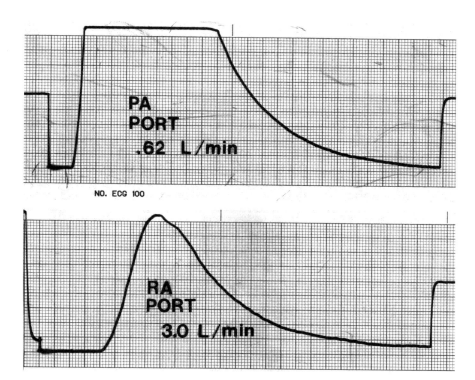

NO. ECG 100

Figure 14.9 Incorrect cardiac output measurement caused by operator error. **Panel A**: This thermodilution curve resulted when iced solution was incorrectly injected through the distal lumen (**PA**). A dramatic decline in pulmonary artery blood temperature was recorded because the thermistor is near the distal lumen. The computer generated cardiac output was 0.62 L/minute. **Panel B**: Correct injection of iced solution through the proximal lumen (**RA port**) generates a normal appearing thermodilution curve in the same patient.

Key Points: Trouble

- A change in the pressure waveform with balloon inflation does not guarantee that a true wedge position has been achieved.

- Many factors can degrade the fidelity of the pressure recording. The causes of a damped tracing include air bubbles, thrombus, catheter kinking and transducer failure.

- Right bundle branch block can occur during catheter insertion and is clinically important in patients with left bundle branch block.

- Examination of the thermodilution cardiac output curve reduces cardiac output measurement error.

Chapter 14 References

1. Matthay MA, Chatterjee K. Bedside catheterization of the pulmonary artery: Risk compared with benefit. *Ann Intern Med* 1988;109:826-834.

2. Foote GA, Schabel SI, Hodges M. Pulmonary complications of the flow-directed balloon-tipped catheter. *N Engl J Med* 1974;290:927-931.

3. Tuman KJ, Carroll GC, Ivankovich AD. Pitfalls in the interpretation of pulmonary artery catheter data. *J Cardiothoracic Anesth* 1989;3:625-641.

4. Gardner RM. Direct blood pressure measurement. Dynamic response requirements. *Anesthesiology* 1981;54:227-236.

5. Barash PG, Nardi D, Hammond G, Walter-Smith G, Capuano D, Laks H, Koprova CJ, Baue AE, Geha AS. Catheter-induced pulmonary artery perforation - mechanisms, management and modification. *J Thorac Cardiovasc Surg* 1981;82:5-12.

6. Sprung CL. Complications of pulmonary artery catheterization. In: Sprung CL, editor. *The Pulmonary Artery Catheter*, 1st ed. Baltimore: University Park Press, 1983;81-84.

7. Sprung CL, Pozen RG, Rozanski JJ, Pinero JR, Eisler BR, Castellanos A. Advanced ventricular arrhythmias during bedside pulmonary artery catheterization. *Am J Med* 1982;72:203-208.

8. Thomson IR, Dalton BC, Lappas DG, Lowenstein E. Right bundle branch block and complete heart block caused by the Swan-Ganz Catheter. *Anesthesiology* 1979;51:359-362.

APPENDIX A: Normal Values

PRESSURES*

Left Ventricle
Systolic	100-140 mmHg
End-diastolic	3-12 mmHg

Right Ventricle
Systolic	15-30 mmHg
End-diastolic	2-8 mmHg

Aortic
Systolic	100-140 mmHg
Diastolic	60-90 mmHg
Mean	70-105 mmHg

Pulmonary Artery
Systolic	15-30 mmHg
Diastolic	4-12 mmHg
Mean	9-18 mmHg

Wedge (left atrium)
Mean	2-12 mmHg
A wave	3-15 mmHg
V wave	3-15 mmHg

Right Atrium
Mean	2-8 mmHg
A wave	2-10 mmHg
V wave	2-10 mmHg

NORMAL VALUES*

Heart Rate (beats/min)	60-100

Resistances (dynes-sec-cm^{-5})

Systemic vascular resistance	700-1600
Total pulmonary resistance	100-300
Pulmonary vascular resistance	20-130

Flow

Cardiac output (L/min)	varies with body surface area
Cardiac Index (L/min/m^2)	2.6 - 4.2
Stroke Index (mL/beat/m^2)	30-65

Oxygen consumption (L/min/m^2)	110-150
Arterial oxygen saturation (%)	93-98
Pulmonary artery (mixed venous) oxygen saturation (%)	75
Arteriovenous oxygen difference (mL/L)	30-50

*Adapted from: Grossman W. Cardiac catheterization and angiography. Philadelphia: Lea & Febiger, 1980:415

APPENDIX B:
Techniques Used in this Book

The hemodynamic data shown in this book were recorded in the George E. Fahr Cardiac Care Unit using a fluid-filled pulmonary artery catheter (Edwards Swan-Ganz, Baxter Healthcare, Irvine, CA, or Opticath, Abbott Laboratories, North Chicago, IL). The distal lumen (pulmonary artery lumen) was connected to a disposable transducer (Medex, Hilliard, Ohio). The proximal lumen (right atrial lumen) was interfaced with the same transducer using a double-stopcock system similar to that described by Civetta. With this system, a single transducer was used to monitor the right atrial, pulmonary artery, and wedge pressure waveforms. The pressure waveform from either the proximal lumen or the distal lumen was easily selected by turning the stopcocks. The dynamic response of the catheter system was tested before insertion by the fast-flash method. Systemic arterial pressures were recorded using a variety of fluid-filled catheters. A four-channel physiologic recorder (Hewlett-Packard, Andover, MA, or Gould, Cleveland, Ohio) was used to simultaneously record the pressure waveform and the single-lead electrocardiogram. A paper speed of 25 mm/sec was usually selected for analysis of the pressure waveforms. A paper speed of 5 or 10 mm/sec was occasionally used to assess the response of intracardiac pressures to respiration or to the hepato-jugular reflux test. Intracardiac pressures were measured at end-expiration because the intrathoracic pressure usually approximates 0 mmHg at this time. The pressure scale was chosen to give an ideal size pressure tracing for visual analysis. For the right atrial pressure, this was usually the 0-25 or 0-30 mmHg scale; for the pulmonary artery pressure and the wedge pressure, the 0-50 or 0-60 mmHg scale; and for the system arterial pressure, the 0-120 or 0-180 mmHg scale. The thermodilution cardiac output was measured using iced D5W solution and a bedside cardiac output computer (Edwards Model 9520, Edwards Laboratories, Santa Ana, CA, or Hewlett-Packard Model 56 Component Monitoring System, Hewlett-Packard, Andover, MA). The thermodilution curves were recorded using a single-channel strip chart recorder.

Subject Index

NOTE: *f* following page numbers indicates figures; *t* indicates tables.